AF322694

# AORTIC SYPHILIS

*Collected Reprints*
*(2009-2022)*

By

WILLIAM C. ROBERTS, MD
and
COLLEAGUES

ISBN: 979-8-88680-084-5
Printed in the United States of America on acid-free paper.

# Preface

If the sinus portion of the ascending aorta is of normal size and the tubular portion of the ascending aorta is diffusely dilated (>5 cm) and neither an acute nor healed aortic dissection is present in the ascending aorta, the diagnosis is usually aortic syphilis. If the intima of the operatively excised aorta is 100% abnormal, the aortic wall is thicker than normal because of diffuse thickening of the intima and adventitia, and focal collections of plasmacytes and lymphocytes are present in the adventitia, a diagnosis of aortic syphilis is confirmed.

Aortic syphilis has not disappeared. It is important to diagnose this condition so that proper antibiotic therapy can be administered in the postoperative period to delay or prevent the occurrence of neurologic syphilis. Often the serologic test for syphilis is negative in patients with aortic syphilis.

—*William C. Roberts, MD*

# Table of Contents



*Articles are numbered based on WCR's CV.

# Natural History of Syphilitic Aortitis

William Clifford Roberts, MD[a,b,*], Jong Mi Ko, BA[a], and Travis James Vowels[a,c]

No large studies of cardiovascular syphilis at necropsy have been reported since 1964. We examined at necropsy 90 patients who had characteristic morphologic findings of syphilitic aortitis. None had ever undergone cardiovascular surgery. With the exception of 2 cases seen more recently, the hearts and aortas of the 90 patients were examined and categorized by one of us (W.C.R.) from 1966 to 1990. All 90 had extensive involvement of the tubular portion of the ascending aorta by the syphilitic process, which spared the sinuses of Valsalva in all but 4 patients. The aortic arch was also involved in 49 (91%) of 54 patients and the descending thoracic aorta in 47 (90%) of 52 patients. Syphilis was the cause of death in 23 (26%) of the 90 patients. It was secondary to rupture of the ascending or descending thoracic aorta in 12, severe aortic regurgitation leading to heart failure in 10, and severe narrowing of the aortic ostium of the right coronary artery in 1 patient. Of the 40 patients who had undergone serologic testing for syphilis, 28 (70%) had a positive (reactive) finding. Those patients with a negative or nonreactive test or who did not undergo a serologic test for syphilis had morphologic and histologic findings in the aorta at necropsy similar to the findings of those patients who had had a positive serologic test for syphilis. In conclusion, cardiovascular syphilis has not disappeared. In patients with dilated ascending aortas, with or without aortic regurgitation, a serologic test for syphilis is recommended. If the findings are positive or if characteristic morphologic features of cardiovascular syphilis are suspected, irrespective of the results of the serologic tests, antibiotic therapy appears desirable.   © 2009 Elsevier Inc. All rights reserved. (Am J Cardiol 2009;104:1578–1587)

Syphilis was so common in the nineteenth century— estimated to affect 15% of United States adults during that period—that an entire specialty (syphilology) focused on it. Although relatively few with primary syphilis subsequently develop tertiary syphilis, the cardiovascular manifestations of late syphilis are at least life-threatening, if not fatal. The cause of the cardiovascular features of syphilis are unclear, because the spirochete *Treponema pallidum* has never convincingly been demonstrated in histologic sections of the aorta in patients with this complication of syphilis, and *T. pallidum* cannot be cultured. Because of its decreased frequency in the past several decades and because serologic tests for syphilis are now infrequently performed, it seemed appropriate to review a large number of cases of cardiovascular syphilis studied at necropsy by a single investigator during an approximately 50-year period to learn more about the morphologic features of the cardiovascular consequences. Only patients who had never undergone cardiovascular surgery were included.

## Methods

The autopsy files of the Pathology Branch of the National Heart, Lung, and Blood Institute, National Institutes of Health (Bethesda, Maryland; where W.C.R. was chief for 29 years) were searched for cases coded as "cardiovascular syphilis." Except for 2 cases seen subsequently, all hearts and aortas were studied by W.C.R. from 1966 through 1990. None of the 90 patients had ever undergone cardiovascular surgery. Of the 90 cases studied, 77 were submitted from Washington, DC area hospitals or institutions (Washington DC Medical Examiners Office, n = 17; Georgetown University Medical Center, n = 17; Washington DC Veterans Affairs Hospital, n = 11; Washington DC General Hospital, n = 12; Howard University Hospital, n = 6; George Washington University Hospital, n = 4; Sibley Memorial Hospital, n = 3; National Institutes of Health, n = 2; Suburban Hospital, n = 2; Franklin Square Hospital, n = 2; National Naval Medical Center, n = 1, and non-Washington, DC area hospitals, n = 13). Patients for whom a serologic test for syphilis was positive (reactive) but in whom the aorta was not involved by the syphilitic process were not included in the present study.

Each heart and aorta was examined initially and later by W.C.R. All hearts had extensive involvement of the tubular portion of the ascending aorta by a process typical of cardiovascular syphilis (to be described subsequently). Many of the hearts and aortas were photographed, and several were drawn by a professional artist (Leon Schlossberg).

Partial or complete clinical records for each case were provided by the submitting institution. Most cases were seen initially by W.C.R. at the submitting institution at a teaching conference. He examined the specimen there and discussed the findings and then brought the heart and aorta back to the National Institutes of Health for additional study. Histologic sections of the aorta and heart were pre-

[a]Baylor Heart and Vascular Institute, Baylor University Medical Center, Dallas, Texas; and [b]Pathology Branch, National Heart, Lung, and Blood Institute, National Institutes of Health, Bethesda, Maryland; [c]University of Texas at Austin, Austin, Texas. Manuscript received July 6, 2009; revised manuscript received and accepted July 6, 2009.

*Corresponding author: Tel: (214) 820-7911; fax: (214) 820-7533.

*E-mail address:* wc.roberts@baylorhealth.edu (W.C. Roberts).

Table 1
Necropsy cases of syphilitic aortitis without operative intervention

| Variable | Total (n = 90) | Men (n = 59) | Women (n = 31) |
|---|---|---|---|
| Age (years) | | | |
| Range | 19–91 | 19–88 (66 ± 13) | 32–91 (70 ± 14) |
| Mean ± SD | 67 ± 14 | | |
| Race | | | |
| African American | 60 | 44 | 16 |
| European American | 20 | 12 | 8 |
| Unclear | 10 | 3 | 7 |
| Serologic test for syphilis (positive/No. done) | 28/40 (70%) | 20/27 (74%) | 8/13 (62%) |
| Aortic regurgitation | 23 (26%) | 14 (24%) | 9 (29%) |
| Systemic hypertension | 41/72 (57%) | 28/48 (58%) | 13/24 (54%) |
| Heart failure | 26/84 (31%) | 23/56 (41%) | 3/28 (11%) |
| Cause of death | | | |
| Syphilis | | | |
| Aortic rupture | 12 (13%) | 5 (8%) | 7 (23%) |
| Aortic regurgitation → heart failure | 10 (11%) | 8 (14%) | 2 (6%) |
| Ostial narrowing, right coronary artery | 1 (1%) | 0 | 1 (3%) |
| Coronary artery disease | 17 (19%) | 14 (24%) | 3 (10%) |
| Stroke | 5 (6%) | 2 (3%) | 3 (10%) |
| Noncardiac, nonvascular | 38 (42%) | 27 (46%) | 11 (35%) |
| Unclear | 7 (8%) | 3 (5%) | 4 (13%) |
| Heart weight (g) | | | |
| Range | 215–850 | 260–850 | 215–750 |
| Mean ± SD | 486 ± 135 | 507 ± 135 | 443 ± 127 |
| Coronary artery narrowing >75% of cross-sectional area | 46/71 (65%) | 35/48 (73%) | 11/23 (48%) |
| Left ventricular infarct | | | |
| Acute | 5 (6%) | 4 (7%) | 1 (3%) |
| Healed | 28 (31%) | 24 (41%) | 4 (13%) |
| Both | 1 (1%) | 0 | 1 (3%) |
| Coronary ostial narrowing | | | |
| Right | 13 (14%) | 9 (15%) | 4 (13%) |
| Left main | 2 (2%) | 1 (2%) | 1 (3%) |

pared at the National Institutes of Health in the Pathology Branch for each case and were examined by W.C.R.

## Results

The pertinent findings for the 59 men and 31 women are listed in Table 1. The men ranged in age from 19 to 88 years (mean 66 ± 13), and the women from 32 to 91 years (mean 70 ± 14). The race was known for 80 patients: 60 (75%) were African American and 20 (25%) were European American. At least 23 patients had some degree of aortic regurgitation; 3 others had evidence of aortic valve stenosis (a nonsyphilitic process) at necropsy. All 90 patients had 3-cuspid aortic valves. At least 41 (57%) of the 72 patients in whom it was noted had a history of systemic hypertension or had had a peak systolic pressure >140 mm Hg or an end-diastolic pressure >90 mm Hg, or both. At least 26 (31%) of the 84 patients in whom it was noted had had clinical evidence of heart failure. At least 40 patients had undergone a serologic test for syphilis (either the Venereal Disease Research Laboratory or fluorescent treponemal antibody), and in ≥28 (70%), 1 or both test results were positive (reactive).

The cause of death in the 90 patients was as follows: cardiovascular syphilis from rupture of the ascending or descending thoracic aorta in 12 patients, severe aortic regurgitation producing heart failure in 10 patients, or severe narrowing of the ostium of the right coronary artery in 1 patient (total 23 patients [26%]); coronary heart disease in 17 patients; stroke in 5 patients; cancer in 14 patients; renal failure in 3 patients; and a noncardiac, nonvascular, and noncancer cause in 28 patients, including chronic obstructive pulmonary disease in 4, amyloidosis in 2, and unclear in 7.

At necropsy, the hearts of the 46 men weighed 260 to 850 g (mean 507 ± 135, median 505). In 33 (72%) of these 46 patients, the heart weighed >400 g (upper limit of normal for men). The hearts of the 23 women weighed 215 to 750 g (mean 443 ± 127, median 420). In ≥18 (78%) of these 23 women, the heart weighed >350 g (upper limit of normal for women).

In all 90 patients, the tubular portion of the ascending aorta was extensively involved by the syphilitic process (Figures 1 to 9). In only 4 of the 90 patients did the process extend into the wall of aorta behind the sinuses of Valsalva. In the other 86 patients, the process began at the sinotubular junction. The aortic arch was available for examination in 54 of the 90 patients. Of the 54 patients, the aortic arch was also involved by the syphilitic process in 49 (91%). The descending thoracic aorta was available for examination in 52 of the 90 patients, and in 47 (90%) the process also involved this portion of the aorta. The abdominal portion of aorta was available for examination in 47 patients, and in 39

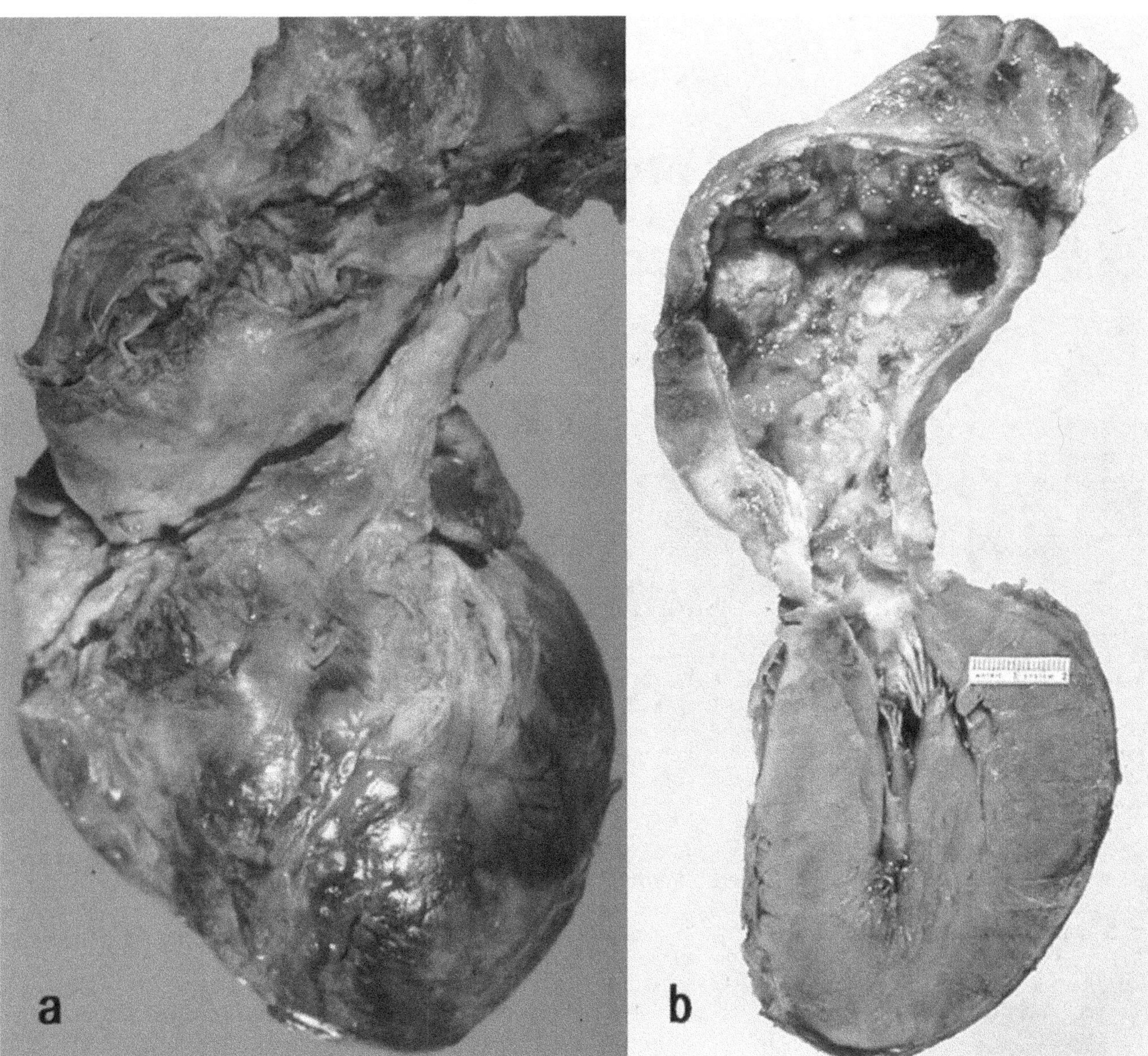

Figure 1. Heart and aorta in 67-year-old European-American woman with positive Venereal Disease Research Laboratory and fluorescent treponemal antibody serologic test results for syphilis with huge fusiform aneurysm of ascending aorta. (*a*) Anterior view of heart and aorta. Huge aortic aneurysm compresses adjacent pulmonary trunk. (*b*) Opened aorta showing severe involvement of tubular portion by syphilitic process with sparing of sinus portion. Right ventricle and atria have been excised from remaining left ventricle. The lack of dilation of the left ventricular cavity strongly suggests the lack of aortic regurgitation, of which no evidence was seen during her life.

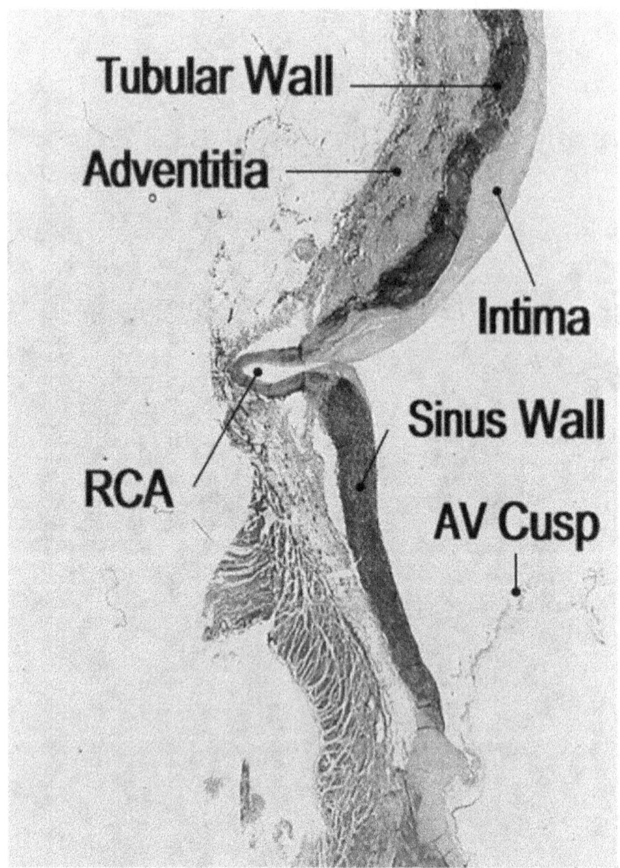


Figure 2. Histologic section of sinus and proximal tubular portion of ascending aorta in 32-year-old African-American woman who was killed in an automotive crash. Ascending aorta had a maximal diameter of 6 cm. Media *(black stained)* of sinus wall was normal, and no intimal or adventitial thickening seen. Wall of tubular portion was 4 times thicker than that of sinus portion. Thickening resulted from severe thickening of both intima and adventitia by fibrous tissue. Transverse scars replaced medial elastic tissue in 3 different areas. Ostium of right coronary artery severely narrowed by intimal fibrous tissue. Movat stain, original magnification ×5. RCA = right coronary artery; AV = aortic valve.

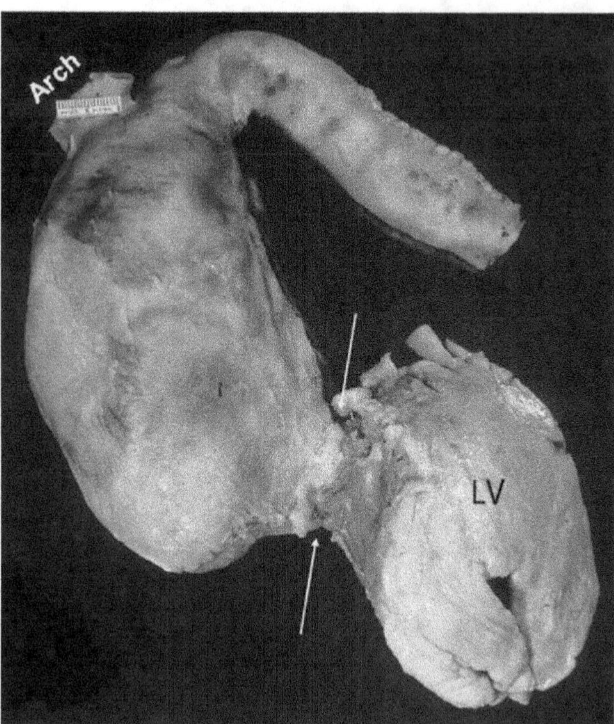


Figure 3. Thoracic aorta and left ventricle from 79-year-old woman who died from cancer. Maximal transverse diameter of ascending aorta was 8.7 cm. Dilation began just above sinus portion *(between arrows)*, which was not dilated. Entire arch and descending thoracic aorta were also diffusely involved by syphilitic process. Both Venereal Disease Research Laboratory and fluorescent treponemal antibody serologic test results for syphilis were negative. LV = left ventricle.

(83%), this portion of the aorta contained atherosclerotic plaques. However, the process was quite different from that involving the more proximal portions of the aorta in that the process involved only the intima and spared the adventitia.

The syphilitic process involving the thoracic aorta caused aneurismal dilation of the involved segment in some patients but not in others. The aneurismal process involved the entire wall of aorta (fusiform) in all patients, and in 10 of them, one or more saccular aneurysms were present within the fusiform dilated portion. (Only a portion of the aortic wall was involved in the saccular aneurysm.)

Histologically, the wall of the thoracic aorta was much thicker than normal, the result of fibrous thickening of the adventitia and fibrous and/or fibrocalcific thickening of the intima (Figures 2 and 8). Within the adventitial fibrous tissue were focal collections of plasmacytes and lymphocytes, often surrounding the vasa vasora, the walls of which were usually quite thickened and their lumens quite narrowed. The media of the aorta was not thickened but its elastic fibers, as demonstrated by Movat stain, were focally interrupted such that in some areas of media no elastic fibers

were present and fibrous scars had replaced the medial elastic fibers and smooth muscle cells. The intimal process appeared to be typical atherosclerotic plaque.

At least 46 (65%) of the 71 patients in whom the arteries were carefully examined had >75% narrowing in the cross-sectional area of one or more major (right, left main, left anterior descending, left circumflex) epicardial coronary arteries. Of the 85 patients in whom the ostia of the 2 coronary arteries in the aorta were carefully examined, 13 (15%) had definite narrowing of the ostium of the right coronary artery and 2 (2%) had definite narrowing of the ostium of the left main coronary artery.

Grossly visible myocardial infarcts were observed at necropsy in 34 (38%) of 89 patients: acute infarcts only in 5 patients (6%), healed infarcts only in 28 patients (31%), and both acute and healed infarcts in 1 patient (1%).

## Discussion

The present study has described the cardiovascular findings at necropsy in 90 patients with characteristic morphologic findings in the ascending aorta of tertiary syphilis. Each heart and aorta was examined and categorized by the same investigator (W.C.R.). No patient had ever undergone cardiovascular surgery. Although it was positive (reactive) for only 70% of the patients who had a serologic test for syphilis, the changes in ascending aorta were similar in the patients with reactive and nonreactive findings for syphilis

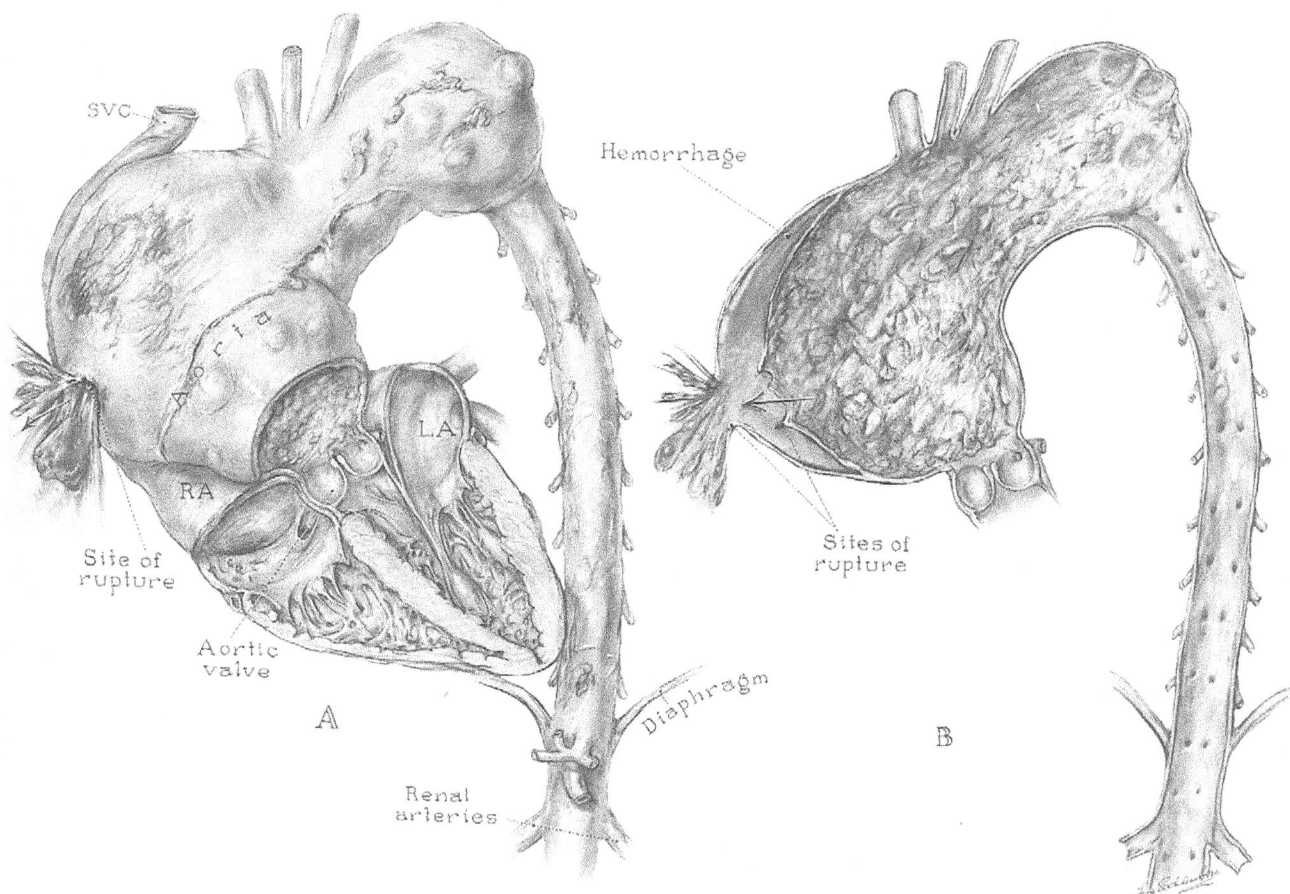


Figure 4. Drawing of thoracic aorta, which ruptured in 60-year-old European-American woman. She had died suddenly at home in the bathroom. Largest transverse diameter of ascending aorta was 9.5 cm. Sinus portion of aorta was normal. The rupture was into the pericardial sac. SVC = Superior vena cava.

and in the patients who did not have a serologic test for syphilis recorded. Of the 90 patients studied, men outnumbered women nearly 2 to 1 and African Americans outnumbered European Americans nearly 3 to 1. Evidence of aortic regurgitation was present clinically in only 1/4 of the patients, and systemic systolic blood pressure >140/90 mm Hg was present in virtually 60% of the patients. Evidence of heart failure was recorded clinically in nearly 1/3 of the patients. The causes of death varied. Syphilis was the cause in only 1/4 of the patients, with nonsyphilitic causes responsible in 3/4. Nearly 70% had one or more major (right, left main, left anterior descending, left circumflex) coronary arteries narrowed >75% in cross-sectional area by atherosclerotic plaques (nonsyphilitic), and nearly 40% of the patients had acute or healed myocardial infarct, or both. The ostium of the right coronary artery was very narrow in 15% of the patients.

Examination of our necropsy patients supports the view that cardiovascular syphilis is essentially limited to the thoracic aorta with occasional involvement of the arch arteries. The involvement when present always included the ascending aorta, but any portion of the thoracic aorta can be affected by the syphilitic process. Although some of our patients had severe atherosclerotic involvement of the abdominal aorta, with or without fusiform aneurysm, the process was clearly different from that involving the thoracic aorta in that it spared the adventitia and only indirectly involved the media (presumably from pressure from the overlying heavy atherosclerotic plaques). Similarly, although the coronary ostia can be narrowed by the syphilitic process in the aorta, the coronary arterial involvement is clearly not a part of the syphilitic process. The narrowing of the coronary arteries themselves resulted from typical atherosclerosis, a process involving the intima only, except for focal thinning of the media, again presumably the result of the overlying heavy atherosclerotic plaques. The adventitia of the coronary arteries was spared (i.e., not thickened).

The syphilitic process appears to involve only arteries in which the vasa vasora are present or at least easily identified histologically. The vasa vasora are either absent from the coronary arteries or difficult to identify. The vasa vasora are present in the entire thoracic aorta but are absent from the abdominal aorta and their absence from this portion of the aorta appears to be the explanation for the absence of syphilitic involvement of the abdominal aorta.

The major consequence of syphilitic involvement of the aorta is thickening of its wall (Figure 10). The thickening results from dense scarring of the adventitia and from less dense fibrous tissue with or without calcium in the intima. The media is not thickened and might be thinner than normal. The media contains many foci of fibrosis, and these scars are usually oriented transversely. In these scarred areas, the elastic fibrils and smooth muscle cells may have vanished completely, and, even in the nonscarred areas of

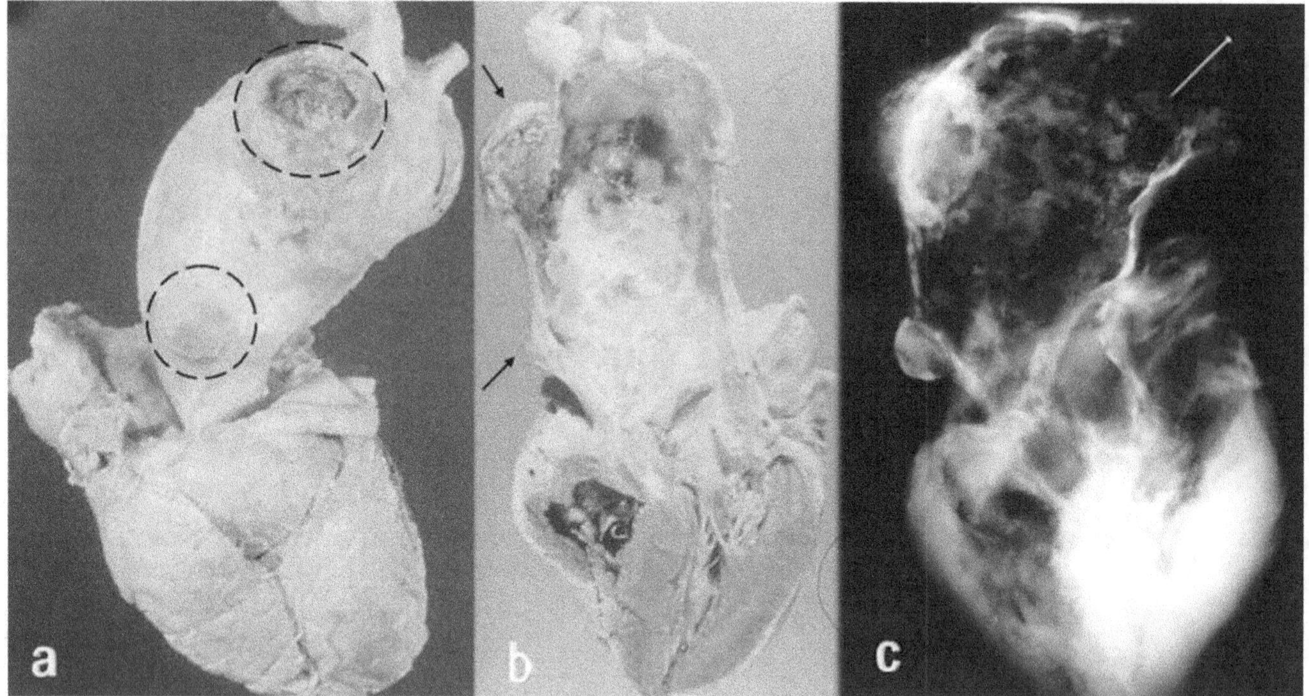

Figure 5. Fusiform and saccular aneurysm of ascending aorta in 81-year-old African-American man who died from a diabetic coma. (*a,b*) One of 2 saccular aneurysms *(arrows and circles)* within fusiform aneurysm had burrowed into the sternum. Thrombus was present in both saccular aneurysms. Sinus portion of aorta was normal. Heart size was normal. (*c*) Calcific deposits present in aortic wall.

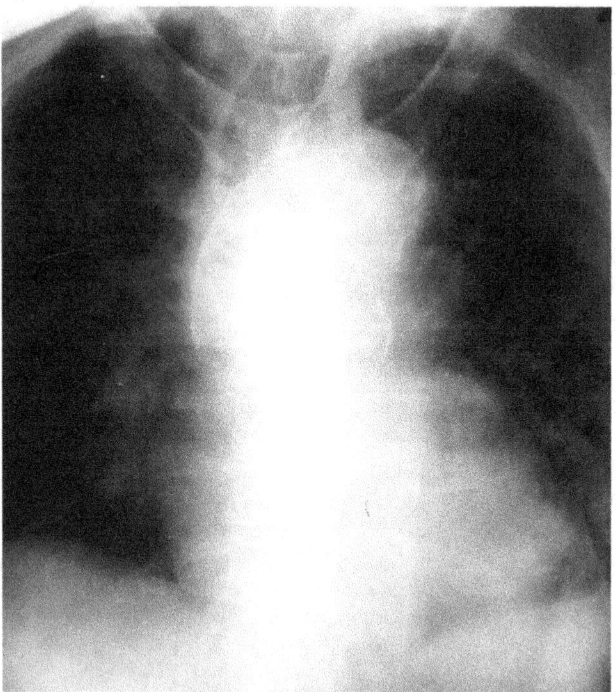

Figure 6. Radiograph of chest in patient described in Figure 5. Linear calcific deposits present in tubular portion of ascending aorta. Calcific deposits present only in intima of aorta.

the media, the elastic fibers are often disrupted. Despite the thickening, the involved arterial wall is weaker than normal because of the disruption of the elastic fibrils and smooth muscle cells of the media. Because the strength of a vessel is dependent on the integrity of its media, which is disrupted, the involved portion of the aorta usually dilates. Where the media has been totally disrupted, the dilation will be particularly severe, resulting in an increase in focal saccular aneurysms.

Accurately reported information on patients in whom cardiovascular syphilis was found at necropsy is relatively limited, primarily because the data obtained was from autopsy protocols and not from examination by the same investigator of a large number of cases or from re-examination by one or more investigators. Clawson and Bell[1] in 1927 reported the findings from necropsy protocols of 126 patients with syphilitic aortitis: 104 (83%) were men and 22 (17%) were women (the ratio of men to women in their total autopsy cases, however, was 2:1). Aortic regurgitation had been evident in 46 patients (37%), rupture of aortic aneurysm occurred in 35 (28%), and myocardial gummas were found in 3 (2%). Sudden death from coronary ostial narrowing occurred in 25 (20%) and the cause of death was nonsyphilitic for 17 (13%).

Martland,[2] in 1930, described necropsy findings from autopsy protocols in 101 patients with morphologic evidence of cardiovascular syphilis: 28 (28%) had ascending aortic aneurysms, 36 (36%) had aortic regurgitation, and 15 (15%) had narrowing of one or more coronary arteries.

Carr,[3] in 1930, briefly described the autopsy findings in 119 patients with morphologic features of cardiovascular syphilis: 13 (11%) had aneurismal dilation of the ascending aorta and 24 (20%) had morphologic evidence of aortic regurgitation; ≥49 patients (41%) had atherosclerotic coronary artery disease.

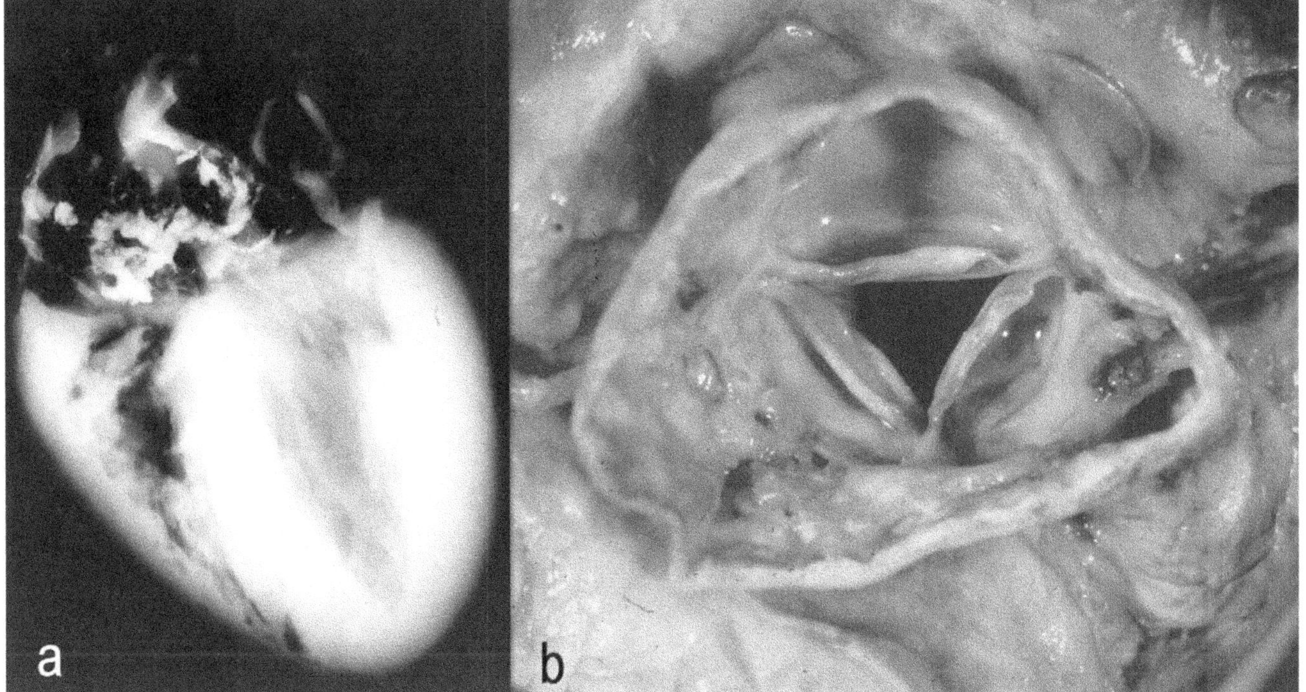

Figure 7. Radiograph of heart and proximal aorta (*a*) at necropsy and of aortic valve and proximal aorta from above (*b*) in 68-year-old African-American woman who had clinical evidence of aortic regurgitation and died from heart failure. Radiograph shows heavy calcific deposits in proximal aorta (*a*). Aortic valve orifice was triangular owing to dilation of ascending aorta. Tubular portion of aorta is diffusely involved by syphilitic process. Venereal Disease Research Laboratory serologic test result for syphilis was nonreactive.

Heggtveit,[4] in 1964, summarized findings from necropsy reports in 100 patients with syphilitic aortitis studied at Kings County Hospital Center (Brooklyn, New York). A clinical diagnosis of syphilis was established in only 17 of the patients. The patients' age range was 30 to 92 years (mean 63): 57 were European American and 43 were African American. Only 23 had ever been treated for syphilis. The blood serology findings (Venereal Disease Research Laboratory and Kolmer) was positive in 40, negative in 28, and not done in 32 patients. Of the 100 patients, 36 had "uncomplicated" aortitis, 40 had aortic aneurysm, 29 had evidence of aortic regurgitation, and 26 had coronary ostial stenosis. In 14 (35%) of the 40 patients with thoracic aortic aneurysms, fatal rupture occurred. In 43 of the 73 men, the heart weighed >400 g and in 18 of the 27 women, the heart weighed >350 g. No large studies of cardiovascular syphilis at necropsy have been reported subsequently.

The frequency of cardiovascular involvement among patients with untreated syphilis has been derived primarily from 2 large studies: the Oslo study and the controversial (i.e., unethical) Tuskegee, Alabama, study, both of which yielded numerous publications in medical journals. The Oslo study[5] analyzed native Oslo patients initially hospitalized with primary syphilis from 1890 to 1910 and followed thereafter for 40 to 60 years. Cardiovascular syphilis (with or without "saccular" thoracic aortic aneurysm, aortic regurgitation or coronary ostial stenosis) was diagnosed in 45 (15%) of the 303 men and in 47 (8%) of the 584 women. Of the patients who were studied at necropsy, 9% of the men had uncomplicated aortitis and 25% had complicated (aneurysm, aortic regurgitation,

coronary ostial stenosis) aortitis, and 11% of the women had "uncomplicated" and 10% had "complicated" disease of the aorta.

The Tuskegee study involved 408 African-American men hospitalized with primary syphilis initially in 1932 and followed through 1972.[6–9] None were treated with penicillin, which had become available in the United States in 1943. By 1952, about 1/3 of the patients had died, and necropsy findings were available for 89. "Fusiform aneurysm of the thoracic aorta" was present in 40 patients (45%), "saccular aneurysm of the thoracic aorta" in 7 (8%), and "aortitis" (by histologic examination) in 41 patients (46%). Of the 89 patients studied at necropsy, 60 (67%) had had positive blood serologic test findings for syphilis when last tested, 3 had "doubtful" test results, and 24 had negative results. Of the 69 hearts (those with weights available), 48 (70%) weighed >400 g. A clinical diagnosis of cardiovascular syphilis corresponded with the necropsy diagnosis in 88% of the patients.

The present study had many limitations. First, we had virtually no information on the presence or absence of primary syphilis in the distant past. Second, the results of the serologic tests for syphilis for most patients were not available to us. Third, the entire aorta of many patients was unavailable for examination by us. Fourth, whether syphilitic cardiovascular disease had been diagnosed clinically was not known for most patients. Finally, the number of patients who had ever received antibiotic therapy for syphilis was unknown to us. Nevertheless, the morphologic data were collected and studied extensively by a single investi-

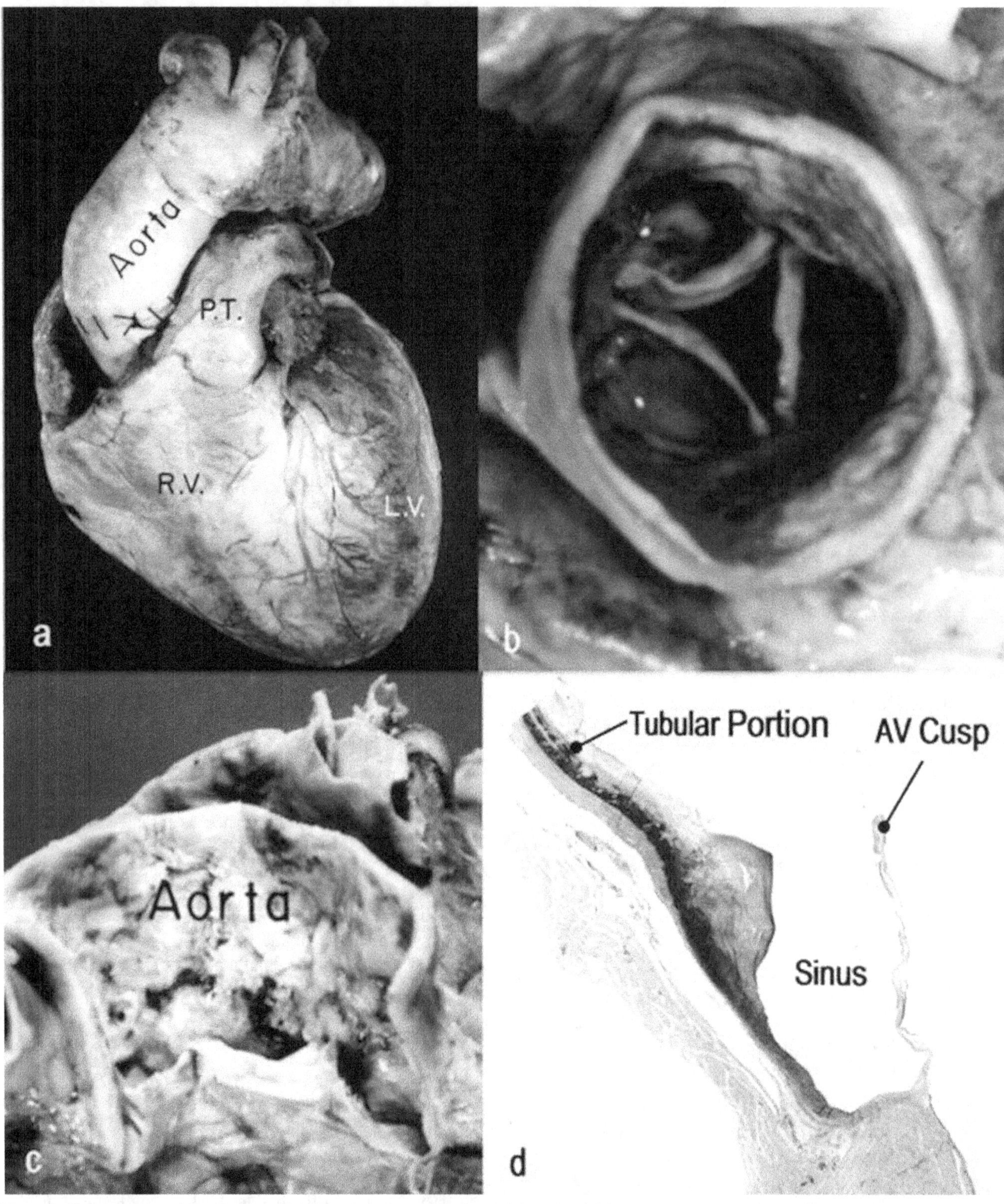


Figure 8. Heart and aorta from 69-year-old African-American man who died from heart failure secondary to severe aortic regurgitation (systemic blood pressure 170/50 mm Hg). Venereal Disease Research Laboratory serologic test result for syphilis was positive (reactive). (*a*) Heart, which weighed 640 g, and dilated ascending aorta. L.V. = left ventricle; P.T. = pulmonary trunk; R.V. = right ventricle. (*b*) Aortic valve from above with eccentric triangular orifice. Wall of aorta was very thick. (*c*) Opened aortic valve and aorta showing diffuse syphilitic involvement of tubular portion. (*d*) Photomicrograph of aortic valve cusp and proximal aorta. Wall behind sinus portion was normal, and wall in tubular portion was about 3 times thicker than aortic wall behind sinus. Elastic van Gieson stain, original magnification ×5.

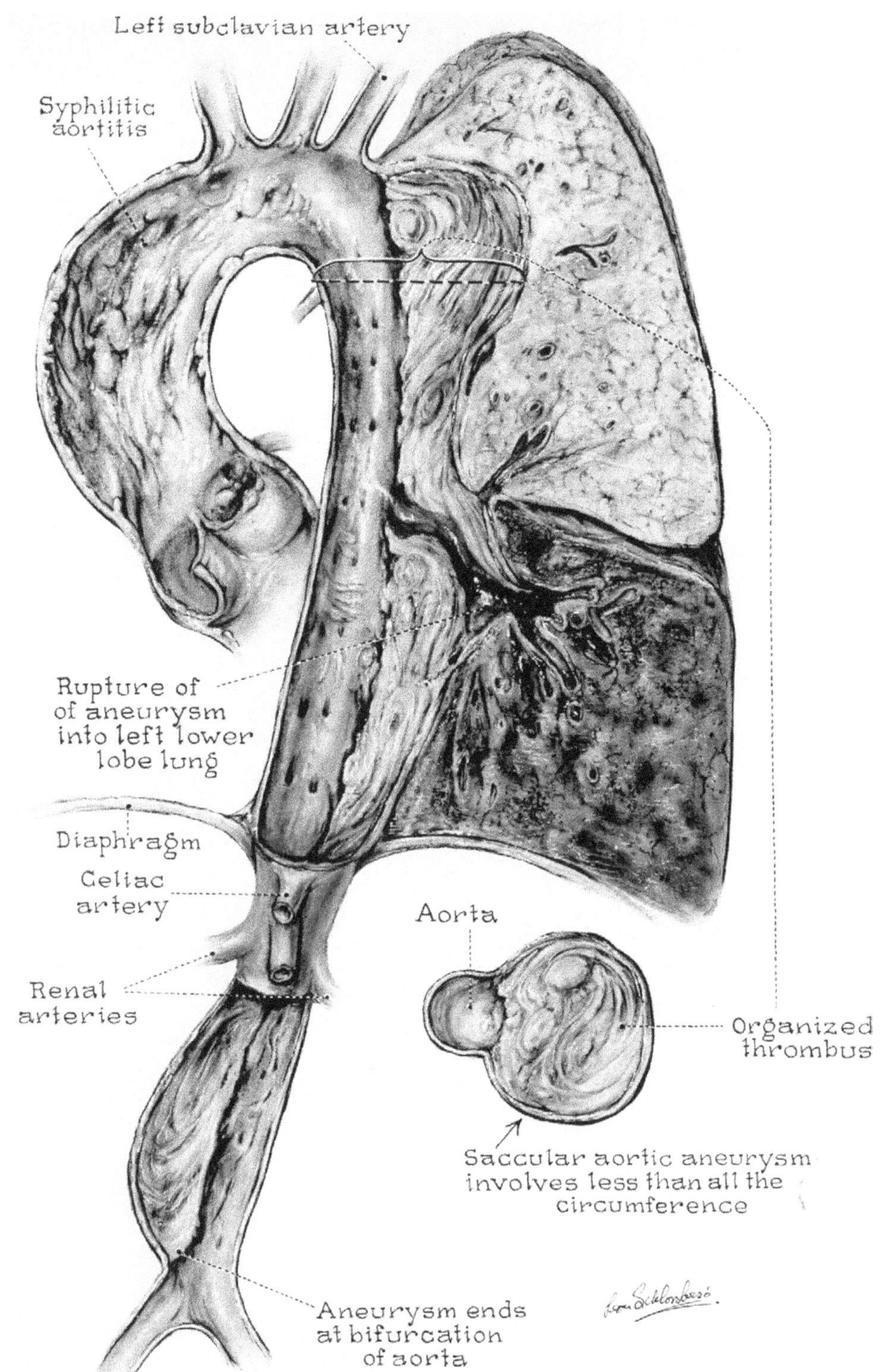


Figure 9. Drawing of aorta and portion of lung from 44-year-old African-American man who died from rupture of descending thoracic aneurysm into his left lung. Ascending aorta was typical of syphilitic aortitis. Wall of aorta behind sinuses was normal. Heart weighed 350 g.

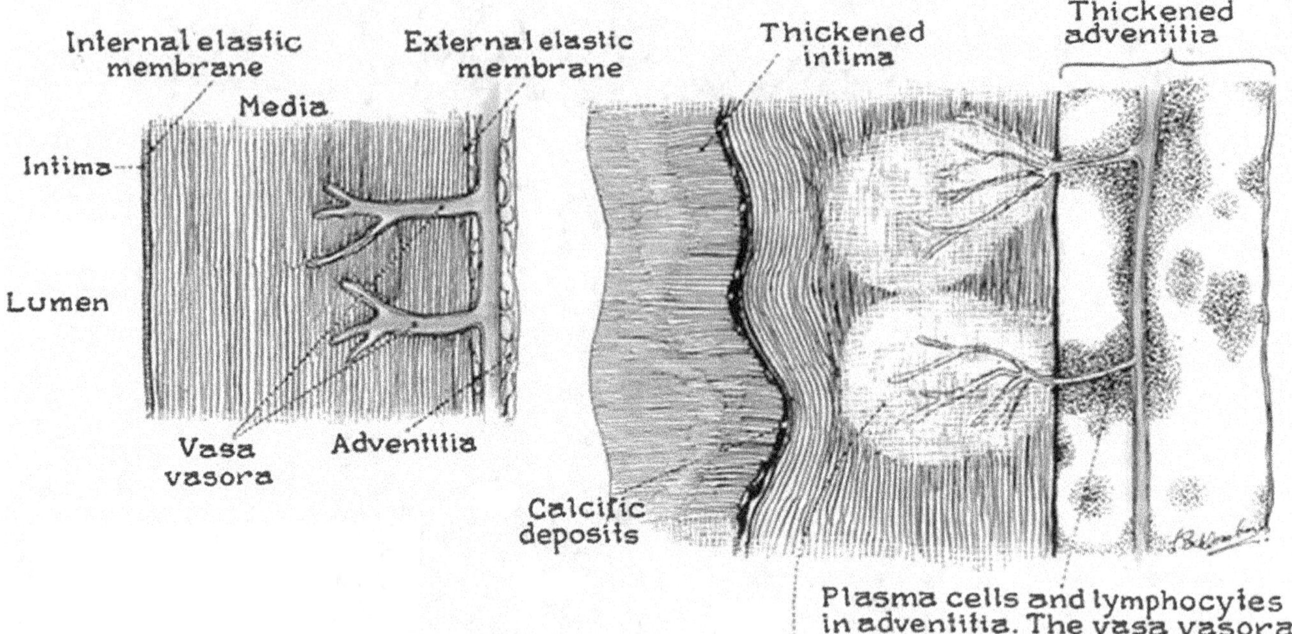


Figure 10. Diagram showing normal aorta *(Left)* and syphilitic aorta *(Right)*.

gator, an occurrence made possible only by not discarding the specimens soon after necropsy.


1. Clawson BJ, Bell ET. The heart in syphilitic aortitis. *Arch Pathol Lab Med* 1927;4:922–936.
2. Martland HS. Symposium on cardiovascular syphilis: syphilis of the aorta and heart. *Am Heart J* 1930;6:1–29.
3. Carr JG. The gross pathology of the heart in cardiovascular syphilis. *Am Heart J* 1930;6:30–36.
4. Heggtveit HA. Syphilitic aortitis: a clinicopathologic autopsy study of 100 cases, 1950 to 1960. *Circulation* 1964;29:346–355.
5. Clark EG, Danbolt N. The Oslo study of the natural history of untreated syphilis: an epidemiologic investigation based on a restudy of the Boeck-Brussgaard material. *J Chronic Dis* 1955;2:311–344.
6. Peters JJ, Peers JH, Olansky S, Cutler JC, Gleeson GA. Untreated syphilis in the male Negro: pathologic findings in syphilitic and nonsyphilitic patients. *J Chronic Dis* 1955;1:127–148.
7. Rockwell DH, Yobs AR, Moore MB Jr. The Tuskegee study of untreated syphilis: the 30th year of observation. *Arch Intern Med* 1964;114:792–798.
8. Caldwell JG, Price EV, Schroeter AL, Fletcher GF. Aortic regurgitation in Tuskegee study of untreated syphilis. *J Chronic Dis* 1973;26:187–194.
9. White RM. Unraveling the Tuskegee study of untreated syphilis. *Arch Intern Med* 2000;160:585–598.

# Identifying Cardiovascular Syphilis at Operation

William Clifford Roberts, MD[a,b,c,*], Rahul Bose, MD[c], Jong Mi Ko, BA[c], Albert Carl Henry, MD[d], and Baron Lloyd Hamman, MD[d]

To describe the morphologic features so the process can be easily identified during surgery, we studied 34 patients with cardiovascular syphilis, 32 of whom underwent excision and replacement of the ascending aorta or aortic valve or both. Of the 34 patients, 22 were treated at Baylor University Medical Center from 1998 to 2008 and 12 at non–Baylor University Medical Center hospitals from 1958 to 1987. In all 34 patients, the tubular portion of the aorta was diffusely thickened and the sinus portion of the aorta was apparently uninvolved. The process involved all 3 layers of the aorta, with thickening of the adventitia, mainly by fibrous tissue. Within the fibrous tissue were collections of plasma cells and lymphocytes, focal destruction of the media without thickening, and marked thickening of the intima by atherosclerotic-appearing lesions. Serologic tests for syphilis were done in only 14 patients (41%) and were positive (reactive) in 6 (43%) of them. The ascending aorta, however, was similar in all 34 patients. In conclusion, cardiovascular syphilis has not disappeared. Its identification during surgery can prompt appropriate antibiotic therapy postoperatively. Although the serologic test results for syphilis might be negative, antibiotic therapy is recommended for patients with panaortitis requiring resection of the ascending aorta with or without aortic regurgitation.    © 2009 Published by Elsevier Inc. (Am J Cardiol 2009;104:1588–1594)

It has been estimated that 15% of men living in the United States in the nineteenth century had syphilis.[1] During the first 60 years of the twentieth century, a serologic test for syphilis was required to obtain a marriage license and was mandatory when admitted to a hospital in the United States. During the past 50 years, however, serologic tests for syphilis have been performed much less frequently than earlier, even in patients with a dilated ascending aorta with or without aortic regurgitation. The morphologic findings of cardiovascular syphilis for the past 100 years have been considered nearly diagnostic of this condition, even when the serologic test result for syphilis has been negative or nonreactive.[2–17] Because the cardiovascular morphologic features of syphilis appear to be underappreciated currently, it seemed appropriate to describe them by focusing on a relatively large group of such patients who underwent surgery for cardiovascular syphilis.

## Methods

A total of 34 patients were analyzed. Of the 34 patients, 10 underwent isolated resection of the tubular portion of the ascending aorta, 6 underwent isolated aortic valve replacement or repair (all later studied at necropsy), 17 underwent both, and 1 underwent resection of an innominate arterial aneurysm with later examination of the entire aorta at necropsy.[18] The criterion for inclusion in the present study was diffuse panaortitis of the tubular portion of the ascending aorta. The diffuseness of involvement was determined by

[a]Department of Internal Medicine, Division of Cardiology, [b]Department of Pathology, [c]Baylor Heart and Vascular Institute, and [d]Department of Cardiothoracic Surgery, Baylor University Medical Center, Dallas, Texas. Manuscript received June 9, 2009; revised manuscript received and accepted June 9, 2009.

*Corresponding author: Tel: (214) 820-7911; fax: (214) 820-7533.

*E-mail address:* wc.roberts@baylorhealth.edu (W.C. Roberts).

gross examination and the panaortitis by histologic examination. Although a rare giant cell might be present in the aorta in the presence of syphilis, giant cell aortitis and Takayasu's arteritis were ruled out by the presence of numerous giant cells in any layer of the aortic wall (intima, media, and adventitia).[19–23] Ankylosing spondylitis[24] was ruled out by the absence of arthritic disease, by the minimal involvement of the ascending aorta, by extension of the process into the sinuses of Valsalva and onto the bases of the aortic valve cusps, and by extension of the process into the anterior mitral leaflet and into the membranous ventricular septum.

All 34 patients had 3-cuspid aortic valves that were free of calcific deposits. The free margins, particularly their central portions were thickened by fibrous tissue in some patients. The dilation of the ascending aorta at surgery was described as involving only its tubular portion, sparing the sinus portion.

A positive or reactive serologic test for syphilis was not considered a criterion for inclusion in the present study, because the test was never done in most patients, or, if performed, the results were unavailable.

All surgically excised aortic valves and ascending aortas and histologic sections of the ascending aorta were examined by one of us (W.C.R.).

## Results

The patients were divided into 2 groups. The first group consisted of 22 patients who underwent surgery at Baylor University Medical Center (BUMC) from 1998 through 2008 (BUMC group). The second group consisted of 12 patients who underwent surgery at 7 non–BUMC hospitals from 1958 to 1987 with examination of the surgically excised tissues and necropsy tissues (10 patients) by one of us (W.C.R.) (non–BUMC group).

The pertinent data for each of the 22 BUMC patients are listed in Table 1. The 15 women were 62 to 82 years old

Table 1

Clinical and morphologic finding for 22 Baylor University Medical Center patients undergoing resection of ascending aorta for cardiovascular syphilis (ascending aortic aneurysm with or without aortic regurgitation)

| Pt. No. | Age (years) at Surgery | Gender | Peak Systolic/End-Diastolic (mm Hg) | | AR (0–4+) | STS Result | BMI (kg/m$^2$) | Year of Surgery | AVR | Aortic Valve Weight (g) | AA Weight (g) | CABG | Interval from Surgery to Death |
|---|---|---|---|---|---|---|---|---|---|---|---|---|---|
| | | | LV | AA | | | | | | | | | |
| 1 | 42 | M | 153/36 | 158/75 | 4+ | R | 23 | 2004 | + | 0.67 | 18 | 0 | NA |
| 2 | 44 | M | — | 120/59* | 0 | R | 25 | 2007 | 0 | NA | — | 0 | 7 days |
| 3 | 51 | M | 109/41 | 119/52 | 4+ | NR | 24 | 2003 | + | 0.58 | 19 | 0 | NA |
| 4 | 59 | M | 143/30 | 139/73 | 3+ | — | 21 | 2003 | + | 0.79 | 21 | 0 | NA |
| 5 | 62 | F | — | 150/—* | 0 | — | 29 | 2008 | 0 | NA | 27 | 0 | 9 days |
| 6 | 64 | M | 100/12 | 107/60 | 4+ | — | 30 | 2004 | 0 | NA | 16 | 0 | NA |
| 7 | 67 | F | 192/33 | 180/69 | 2+ | — | 21 | 2003 | + | 0.76 | 19 | + | NA |
| 8 | 69 | F | 99/7 | 95/44 | 0 | — | 27 | 2004 | 0 | NA | 22 | 0 | NA |
| 9 | 69 | M | 161/11 | 171/66 | 3+ | — | 25 | 2005 | + | 0.63 | 25 | + | 21 days |
| 10 | 71 | M | — | 100/58 | 0 | — | 20 | 1998 | 0 | NA | 44 | + | 179 days |
| 11 | 71 | F | — | 146/44* | 4+ | — | 28 | 1998 | + | — | 10 | 0 | 42 days |
| 12 | 71 | F | — | 154/70* | 1+ | — | 29 | 2005 | + | 0.45 | 16 | 0 | NA |
| 13 | 71 | F | 135/12 | 153/70 | 4+ | NR | 31 | 2007 | + | 0.64 | 40 | + | NA |
| 14 | 72 | F | — | — | +† | — | 22 | 2000 | +† | 0.35 | 16 | + | 0 (OR) |
| 15 | 73 | F | 138/17 | 139/65 | 0 | — | 27 | 2005 | 0 | NA | 19 | + | NA |
| 16 | 75 | F | 124/0 | 104/30 | 3+ | — | 26 | 2006 | + | 0.56 | 18 | + | NA |
| 17 | 75 | F | 141/17 | 148/71 | 0 | — | 18 | 2006 | 0 | NA | 19 | 0 | NA |
| 18 | 75 | F | 123/28 | 112/42 | 1+ | NR | 21 | 2008 | 0 | NA | 21 | + | NA |
| 19 | 78 | F | — | 182/55 | 3+ | — | 27 | 2008 | + | 0.78 | 26 | 0 | 25 days |
| 20 | 79 | F | 138/8 | 145/52 | +† | — | 22 | 1999 | + | 0.40 | 21 | 0 | 23 days |
| 21 | 81 | F | — | 150/60* | +† | — | 27 | 1999 | + | 0.70 | 1 | + | 2 years |
| 22 | 82 | F | 151/15 | 146/57 | 3+ | — | 30 | 2001 | + | 0.59 | 9 | 0 | NA |

* Indirect pressure.

† Degree of AR unclear.

AA = ascending aorta; AR = aortic regurgitation; AVR = aortic valve replacement; BMI = body mass index; CABG = coronary artery bypass grafting; F = female; LV = left ventricular; M = male; NA = not applicable; NR = nonreactive; OR = operating room; Pt. No. = patient number; R = reactive; RCA = right coronary artery; STS = serologic test for syphilis; — = no information available.

Table 2

Clinical and morphologic finding in 12 non–Baylor University Medical Center patients undergoing cardiovascular surgery for cardiac syphilis (ascending aortic aneurysm with or without aortic regurgitation)

| Pt. No. | Age (years) at Surgery | Gender | Peak Systolic/End-Diastolic (mm Hg) | | AR (0–4+) | Narrowed Ostium RCA | CAD | STS Result | Year of Surgery | AVR | Prosthesis Type | AA Resected | Interval from Surgery to Death | HW (g) |
|---|---|---|---|---|---|---|---|---|---|---|---|---|---|---|
| | | | LV | AA | | | | | | | | | | |
| 1 | 37 | M | 160/20 | 160/35 | 4+ | + | + | NR | 1961 | 0* | NA | 0 | 0 (OR) | 600 |
| 2 | 49 | F | — | 180/70† | 4+ | 0 | 0 | R | 1958 | 0‡ | NA | +§ | 19 years | — |
| 3 | 49 | M | 130/35 | 130/60 | 3+ | — | 0 | NR | 1983 | + | Prosthesis | + | — | — |
| 4 | 50 | M | — | 160/50† | 1+ | + | 0 | R | 1970 | 0 | NA | + | 0 (OR) | 700 |
| 5 | 53 | M | 143/18 | 152/40 | 4+ | 0 | 0 | R | 1965 | + | S-E | 0 | 13 days | 600 |
| 6 | 54 | M | — | 140/50 | 4+ | 0 | 0 | NR | 1980 | + | B-S | 0‖ | 0 (OR) | 740 |
| 7 | 56 | F | 106/25 | 108/27 | 4+ | + | + | NR | 1964 | + | S-E | + | 2 days | 800 |
| 8 | 60 | F | — | 200/110¶ | +# | — | 0 | — | 1987 | + | Prosthesis | + | 4 years | 360 |
| 9 | 61 | F | — | — | +# | + | 0 | — | 1985 | + | Porcine | 0 | 8 years | 700 |
| 10 | 63 | M | 150/8 | 160/60 | +# | 0 | 0 | — | 1972 | + | B-S | + | 8 years | 790 |
| 11 | 65 | F | 120/8 | 120/65 | +# | — | 0 | NR | 1979 | + | Porcine | + | 0 (OR) | — |
| 12 | 65 | F | 170/8 | 180/50 | 4+ | + | + | R | 1977 | + | Porcine | 0 | 6 hours | 700 |

* Aortic valve repair.

† Indirect pressure.

‡ Hufnagel prosthesis placed in descending thoracic aorta.

§ AA resected at third operation.

‖ AA was wrapped.

¶ History of high blood pressure found in autopsy report.

# Degree of AR unclear.

AA = ascending aorta; AVR = aortic valve replacement; B-S = Bjork-Shiley; CAD = coronary artery disease; F = female; HW = heart weight; LV = left ventricular; M = male; NA = not applicable; NR = nonreactive; Op = operation; OR = operating room; R = reactive; RCA = right coronary artery; S-E = Starr-Edwards; STS = serologic test for syphilis; — = no information available.

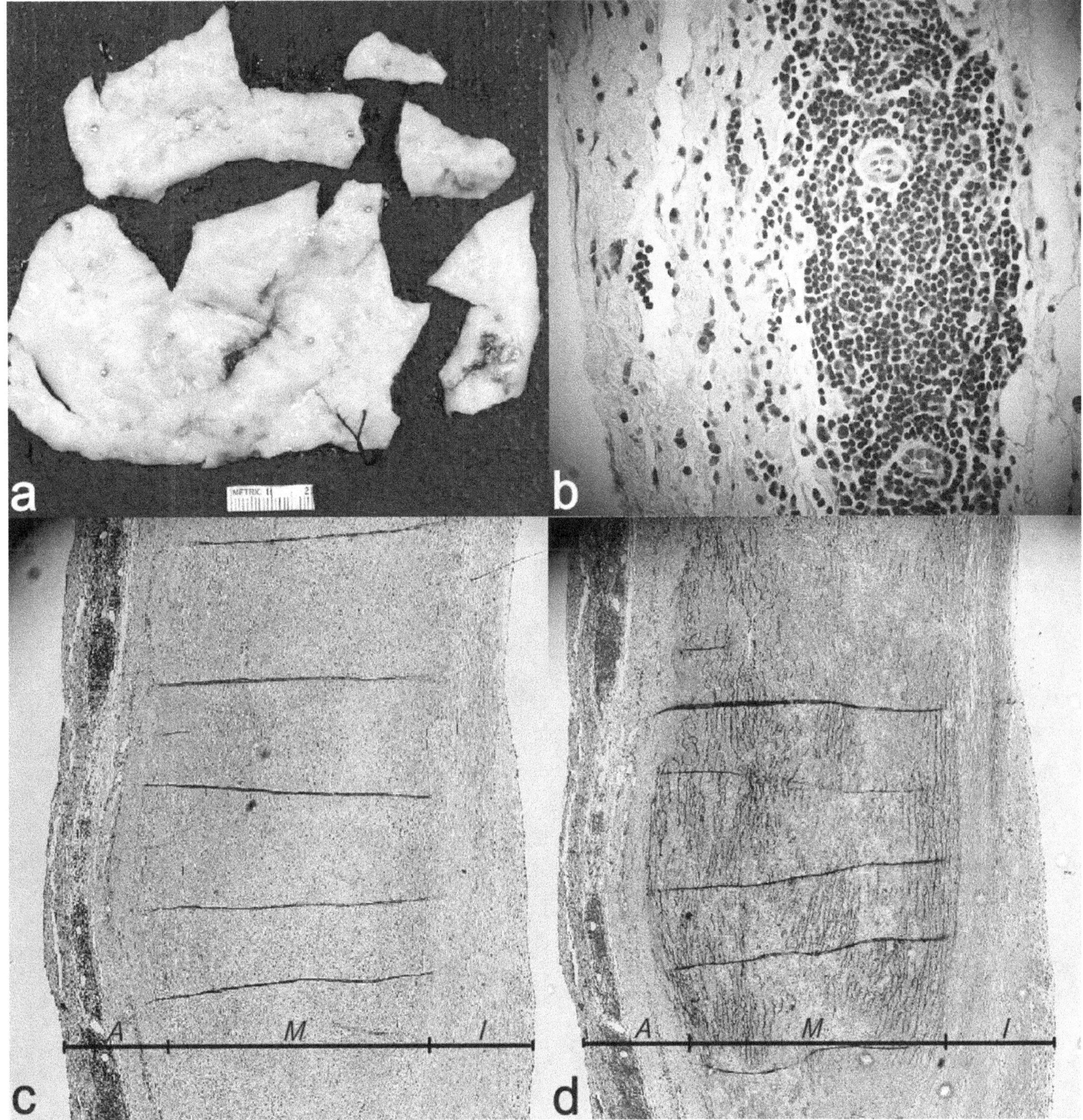

Figure 1. Patient 5 in Table 1. *(a)* Portion of tubular portion of ascending aorta removed at surgery. Ascending aorta preoperatively had 7.0-cm in diameter. Every square millimeter of intimal surface was abnormal. *(b)* Close-up of collection of plasma cells and lymphocytes in adventitia. Hematoxylin and eosin stain, original magnification ×400. *(c,d)* Through-and-through thickness of aorta at same site but with different stains: *(c)* hematoxylin and eosin stain and *(d)* Movat's stain. A = adventitia; M = media; I = intima. Adventitia contained several collections of plasmacytes and lymphocytes. *(d)* Stain showing marked interruption of medial elastic fibers. *(c, d)* Original magnification ×40.

(mean 73), and the 7 men were 42 to 71 years old (mean 57). The degree of aortic regurgitation varied from 0 to 4+/4+, and 14 (64%) had replacement of the aortic valve, which varied in weight from 0.35 to 0.79 g (mean 0.61). (The normal aortic valve weight is about 0.50 g.[25]) Portions of the ascending aorta were resected in all 22 patients. Excluding the 1 patient who only underwent biopsy of the aorta (patient 21), the weight of the resected aortas was 9 to

44 g (mean 23 g for the 7 men and 20 g for the 14 women). On coronary angiography, 9 (41%) of the 22 patients had >50% narrowing in the diameter of one or more major epicardial coronary arteries, and all underwent concomitant coronary artery bypass grafting.

The pertinent data for each of the 12 non–BUMC patients are summarized in Table 2. The 6 women were 49 to 65 years old (mean 59), and the 6 men were 37 to 63 years

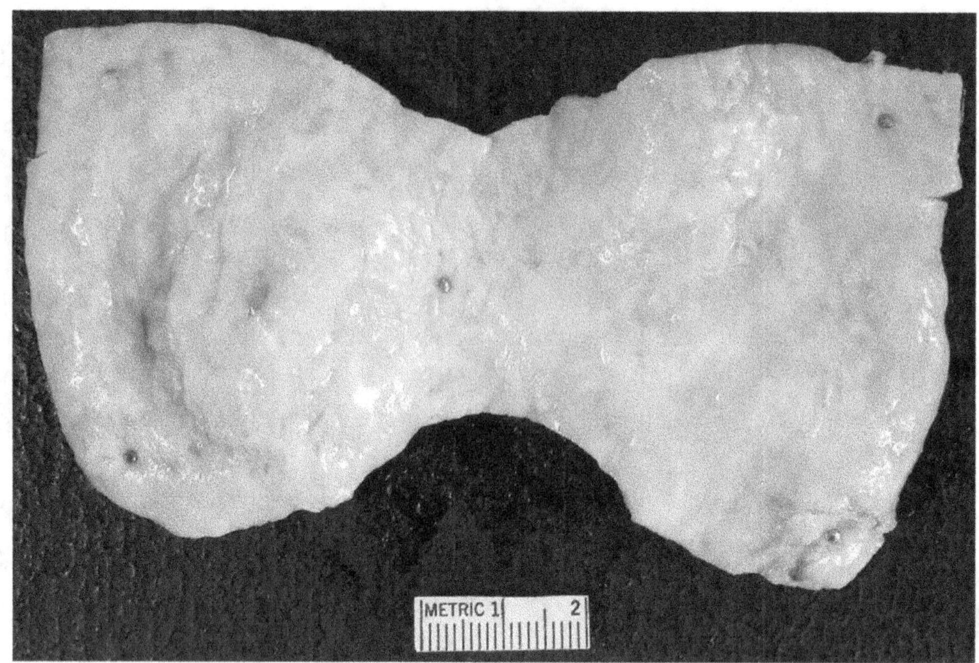

Figure 2. Patient 18 in Table 1. Portion of ascending aorta resected at surgery. Every square millimeter diffusely involved. Preoperative ascending aorta had 5.6-cm in diameter.

old (mean 51). All 12 had some degree of aortic regurgitation, usually severe, and aortic valve replacement (n = 9) or repair (n = 1) was performed in 10 (92%). Portions of the ascending aorta were resected in 7 patients (58%), and it was "wrapped" in 1 patient (8%). Of the 5 patients in whom portions of the ascending aorta were not resected during surgery, all subsequently died (3 within 2 weeks of surgery). The aorta from each of these 5 patients was examined at autopsy by one of us (W.C.R.). At least 11 of the 12 patients died (no information was available for 1 patient). Of the 11 patients, 7 died within 2 weeks of surgery and 4 died later. Of the 4 latter patients, 2 died at reoperation (one procedure to repair a parabasilar leak and the other to excise the prosthesis in the descending aorta), 1 patient died in an auto accident, and 1 died from gangrenous bowel after surgery. An autopsy was performed in each. Calcific deposits were present and extensive in the ascending aorta in all 12 patients. The ostium of the right coronary artery was narrowed considerably in ≥5 of the 12 patients. More than 75% narrowing in the cross-sectional area was present in one or more major coronary arteries in 3 of the 12 patients (determined by angiography or autopsy).

A serologic test for syphilis was performed preoperatively for 5 of the 22 BUMC patients, and 2 results were positive. The test was performed for 9 of the 12 non–BUMC patients, and 4 results were positive (reactive) and 5 negative (nonreactive).

## Discussion

In ≥26 of the 34 patients reported, a diagnosis of cardiovascular syphilis was not suspected clinically or during surgery. The diagnosis was not made until examination of the surgically excised ascending aorta in 28 patients or at necropsy in 6 patients. In each case, the sinus portion of the aorta was spared, and the process involved only the tubular portion of ascending aorta with or without some involvement of the arteries arising from the aortic arch. One patient (patient 2; Table 1) had a syphilitic aneurysm of the innominate artery, in addition to involvement of the ascending, transverse, and descending portions of the aorta.[18]

The involvement of the ascending aorta in all cases was diffuse, meaning that it involved virtually every square millimeter of the ascending aorta, beginning at the junction of the sinus portion and the tubular portion of the ascending aorta (Figures 1 to 4). Histologically, all 3 layers of the aorta were involved (Figures 1 and 3). The adventitia was thickened mainly by fibrous tissue within which were thickened and narrowed vasa vasora vessels surrounded by collections of plasma cells and lymphocytes. Elastic stains of the aortic wall disclosed transverse scars in the media resulting in focal, but extensive, loss of the medial elastic fibers and replacement by fibrous tissue. The medial smooth muscle cells were also replaced by fibrous tissue. The intima in all cases was thickened by what appeared to be typical atherosclerotic plaque. This process resulted in a thickened aortic wall caused by thickening of the adventitia and intima. Although the media was greatly abnormal, it was not thickened.

Thus, the key to recognizing cardiovascular syphilis during surgery is the diffuse nature of the involvement of the tubular portion of the ascending aorta with complete or virtually complete sparing of the sinus portion of the aorta. Focal saccular aneurysm can occur in the tubular portion of the aorta, in addition to the diffuse dilation of the ascending aorta.

Although the wall of aorta is thicker than normal in the presence of cardiovascular syphilis, it is nevertheless weaker than normal because the integrity of the media has

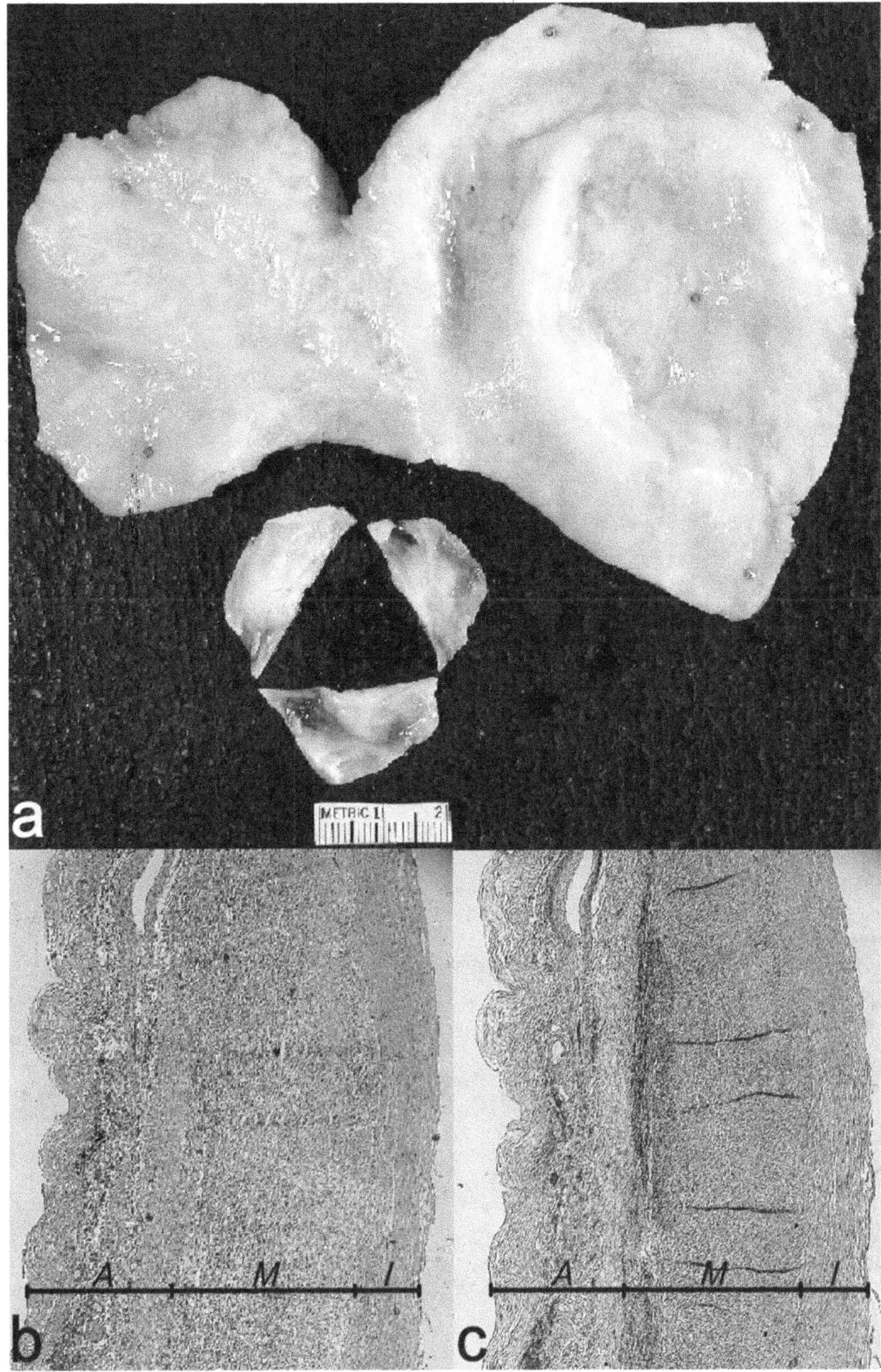

Figure 3. Patient 19 in Table 1. *(a)* Operatively excised ascending aorta and aortic valve. Ascending aorta preoperatively had maximal diameter of 6.5 cm. Every square millimeter of intimal surface of aorta was abnormal. Narrow portion of aorta represents its left border and wide diameter, its right border. Three-cuspid aortic valve normal for age of patient. *(b, c)* Photomicrographs of same portion of aorta. A = adventitia; M = media; I = intima. Most elastic fibers *(stained black)* in media have disappeared. Inflammatory cells are present in thickened adventitia. Hematoxylin and eosin stain *(b)* and Movat's stain *(c)*; original magnification for each ×40.

been interrupted by transverse scars. Therefore, the aorta usually dilates. This could be the cardiovascular paradox of syphilis in that the aortic wall, although thicker than normal, is weaker than normal.

One condition grossly similar to cardiovascular syphilis is *giant cell arteritis*.[20] This process, however, can also involve the sinus portion of the aorta and the arteries arising from the aorta. However, histologically, many large giant

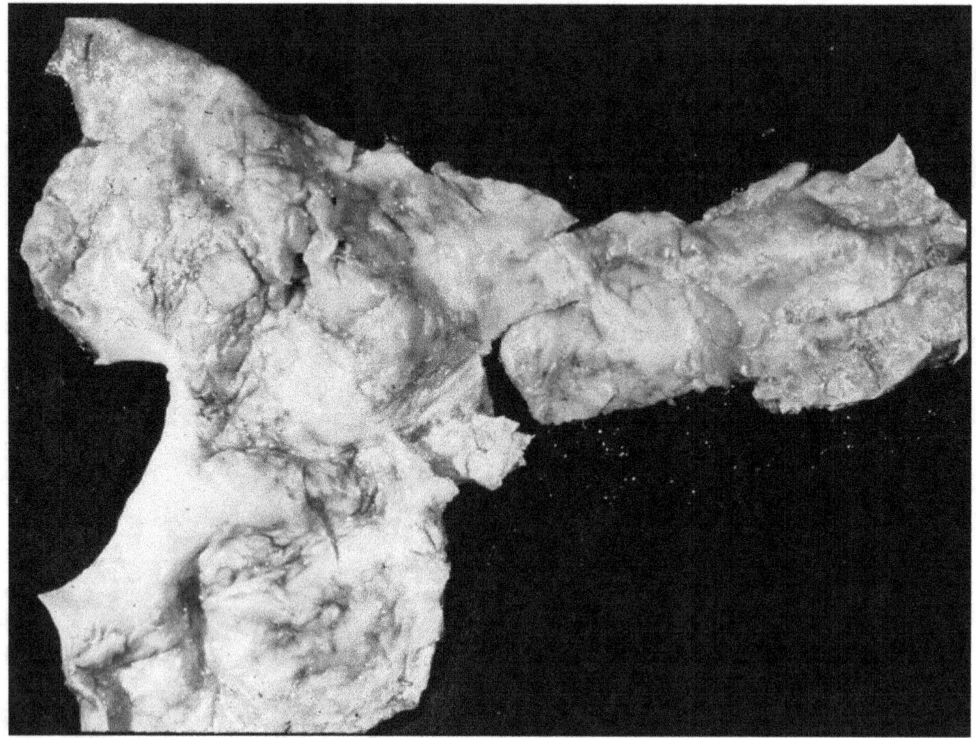

Figure 4. Patient 7 in Table 2. Operatively excised ascending aorta totally involved except for small portion on left, which probably represents wall of sinus portion of aorta. Numerous calcific deposits are present and located in intima.

cells are present in the aortic wall. In contrast, giant cells are absent or virtually absent in the aorta in patients with cardiovascular syphilis.

*Ankylosing spondylitis* can also resemble cardiovascular syphilis histologically; however, its distribution is entirely different from that of cardiovascular syphilis.[24] Ankylosing spondylitis involves the wall of the sinus portion of the aorta, the aortic valve, and extends into the anterior mitral leaflet and the membranous portion of the ventricular septum. Such extension into the aortic valve (mainly its bases—near the site of attachment of the cusps) and caudal to the valve never occurs in cardiovascular syphilis. As a result, heart block (left bundle branch block or complete heart block) is common in patients with ankylosing spondylitis but is usually absent in those with cardiovascular syphilis. If it is present in patients with cardiovascular syphilis, it is not the result of that process. Also, in ankylosing spondylitis, the process extends only 1 cm or so into the tubular portion of the ascending aorta. Most of these patients also have the HLA-B27 gene.

The reason the serologic test result for syphilis is positive (reactive) in some patients with syphilitic aortitis and negative (nonreactive) in others is unknown.[26] The morphologic features of cardiovascular syphilis appear to be more specific for this condition than the serologic test.

The major limitation of the present study was the absence of positive or reactive serologic test results for syphilis for most of the patients. Of the 22 BUMC patients, 17 never had a serologic test for syphilis performed. Of the 5 who did, only 2 had positive or reactive results. Nevertheless, the gross and histologic features of the ascending aorta were both similar in the patients with and without serologic

tests performed and in the few with and without positive serology.

Another potential weakness was that the sinus portion of aorta was examined in only the 13 patients who were studied at necropsy after cardiovascular surgery by one of us (W.C.R.). In all of 13, the aortic wall behind the sinuses was of normal thickness.


1. Hayden D. Pox: Genius, Madness, and the Mysteries of Syphilis. New York: Basic Books, 2003.
2. Cowan J, Rennie JK. Syphilis of the heart. *BMJ* 1921;2:184–186.
3. Clawson BJ, Bell ET. The heart in syphilitic aortitis. *Arch Pathol Lab Med* 1927;4:922–936.
4. Martland HS. Symposium on cardiovascular syphilis: syphilis of the aorta and heart. *Am Heart J* 1930;6:1–29.
5. Reid WD. The diagnosis of cardiovascular syphilis; analysis of clinical and postmortem findings. *Am Heart J* 1930;6:91–106.
6. Welty JW. A necropsy survey of cardiovascular syphilis with particular reference to its decreasing incidence. *Am J Med Sci* 1939;197:782–793.
7. Nichols CF. A study of syphilis of the aorta and aortic valve area. *Ann Intern Med* 1940;14:960–976.
8. Levitt A, Levy DS. Syphilitic aortic disease: an analysis of 508 cases. *NY State J Med* 1940;40:648–652.
9. Thorner MC, Carter RA, Griffith GC. Calcification as a diagnostic sign of syphilitic aortitis. *Am Heart J* 1949;38:641–653.
10. Clawson BJ. Syphilitic cardiac deaths in over fifty thousand autopsies. *Minn Med* 1950;33:437–440.
11. Webster B, Rich C Jr, Densen PM, Moore JE, Nicol CS, Padget P. Studies in cardiovascular syphilis. III. The natural history of syphilitic aortic insufficiency. *Am Heart J* 1953;46:117–145.
12. Peters JJ, Peers JH, Olansky S, Cutler JC, Gleeson GA. Untreated syphilis in the male Negro; pathologic findings in syphilitic and nonsyphilitic patients. *J Chronic Dis* 1955;1:127–148.
13. Halpert B, Willms RK. Aneurysms of the aorta: an analysis of 249 necropsies. *Arch Pathol* 1962;74:163–168.

14. Heggtveit HA. Syphilitic aortitis: a clinicopathologic autopsy study of 100 cases, 1950 to 1960. *Circulation* 1964;29:346–355.
15. Levine SA. The diagnosis of syphilitic aortitis with negative Wassermann reactions. *Am Heart J* 1930;6:116–120.
16. Beckh W. The serologic reaction in cardiovascular syphilis. *Am Heart J* 1943;25:307–312.
17. Jackman JD Jr, Radolf JD. Cardiovascular syphilis. *Am J Med* 1989;87:425–433.
18. Roberts WC, Kourlis H Jr, Ko JM, Newberry J, Burton E, Hebeler RF Jr. Full-blown syphilis with aneurysm of the innominate artery. *Am J Cardiol* 2009, in press.
19. Roberts WC, MacGregor RR, DeBlanc HJ Jr, Beiser GD, Wolff SM. The prepulseless phase of pulseless disease, or pulseless disease with pulses. A newly recognized cause of cardiac disease, monoclonal gammopathy and "fever of unknown origin." *Am J Med* 1969;46:313–324.
20. Honig HS, Weintraub AM, Gomes MN, Hufnagel CA, Roberts WC. Severe aortic regurgitation secondary to idiopathic aortitis. *Am J Med* 1977;63:623–633.
21. Tavora F, Burke A. Review of isolated ascending aortitis: differential diagnosis, including syphilitic, Takayasu's and giant cell aortitis. *Pathology* 2006;38:302–308.
22. Miller DV, Isotalo PA, Weyand CM, Edwards WD, Aubry M-C, Tazelaar HD. Surgical pathology of noninfectious ascending aortitis: a study of 45 cases with emphasis on an isolated variant. *Am J Surg Pathol* 2006;30:1150–1158.
23. Homme JL, Aubry M-C, Edwards WD, Bagniewski SM, Shane Pankratz V, Kral CA, Tazelaar HD. Surgical pathology of the ascending aorta: a clinicopathologic study of 513 cases. *Am J Surg Pathol* 2006;30:1159–1168.
24. Bulkley BH, Roberts WC. Ankylosing spondylitis and aortic regurgitation: description of the characteristic cardiovascular lesion from study of eight necropsy patients. *Circulation* 1973;48:1014–1027.
25. Silver MA, Roberts WC. Detailed anatomy of the normally functioning aortic valve in hearts of normal and increased weight. *Am J Cardiol* 1985;55:454–461.
26. Ratnam S. The laboratory diagnosis of syphilis. *Can J Infect Dis Med Microbiol* 2005;16:45–51.

# Full Blown Cardiovascular Syphilis with Aneurysm of the Innominate Artery

William Clifford Roberts, MD[a,b,c,]*, Forrester Dubus Lensing, MD[d], Harry Kourlis, Jr., MD[e], Jong Mi Ko, BA[c], Jonathan Warren Newberry, MD[b], Michael John Smerud, MD[d], Elizabeth C. Burton, MD[b], and Robert Frederick Hebeler, Jr., MD[e]

The investigators report the case of a 44-year-old man who presented acutely and was found to have saccular aneurysm of the innominate artery, narrowed or totally occluded aortic arch arteries, and marked thickening of the thoracic aorta except for the wall behind the sinuses of Valsalva. The abdominal aorta was entirely normal. Results of the serologic test for syphilis were strongly positive. Because cardiovascular syphilis appears to be a disease that affects the vasa vasora and because these channels are limited to the thoracic aorta, the abdominal aorta is uninvolved, as demonstrated so nicely in the patient described in this case report. Because most patients with cardiovascular syphilis are much older than the patient described, it is unusual to see a perfectly normal abdominal aorta, as in the present patient. In conclusion, syphilis producing aneurysm of the innominate artery is unusual but is always associated with syphilitic involvement of the thoracic aorta.   © 2009 Elsevier Inc. All rights reserved. (Am J Cardiol 2009;104:1595–1600)

Recently, we studied a young man who presented with evidence of a saccular aneurysm of the innominate artery and narrowing or total occlusions of the arteries from the aortic arch. Operative resection of the aneurysm and bypassing of the 2 obstructed arteries, although initially successful, proved to be unsuccessful, and the entire thoracic aorta and its major branches were found to be affected by cardiovascular syphilis. Because of the unusual opportunity to study the morphologic features of full-blown cardiovascular syphilis in a relatively young patient, and because of the presence of a saccular aneurysm of an arch artery, the present case is described.

## Case Description

A 44-year-old white man born in February 1963 had been in his usual health except for right-hand claudication when doing hard labor until September 2007, when he developed substernal chest pain and fainted. He was brought to his local hospital and found to have marked differences in the pulses in the arms, and because of the possibility of aortic dissection, he was transferred to Baylor University Medical Center.

Computed tomographic angiographic examination (Figure 1) on admission showed a 5.6-cm saccular aneurysm of the innominate artery, severe narrowing of the right common carotid and vertebral arteries and the celiac axis at their origins, and totally occluded left common carotid and left subclavian arteries. The right subclavian and left vertebral arteries were patent. The wall of the entire thoracic aorta, except for the wall behind the aortic sinuses, was thick-

ened. A 3-dimensional reconstruction best demonstrated the saccular aneurysm of the innominate artery (Figure 2). Gadolinium-enhanced magnetic resonance angiography (Figure 3) better showed the intracerebral and extracerebral blow flow.

Although the results of the Venereal Disease Research Laboratory test for syphilis were nonreactive, the results of rapid plasma reagin were positive ($>$1:512), and the treponema palladium particle agglutination was also reactive. Antinuclear antibodies were present, and in titer 1 they were 1:2,560, and strong cytoplasmic speckling was noted. The C-reactive protein level was 8.9 mg/dl, and the erythrocyte sedimentation rate was 105 mm/hour. The results of cerebrospinal fluid test for syphilis (rapid plasma reagin) were negative.

At operation in September 2007, the aneurysm was excised, Dacron grafts were placed from the aorta to the right and left common carotid arteries, and a saphenous vein graft was placed from the Dacron graft to the right vertebral artery. The 7-day postoperative course initially was smooth, but the patient's last 2 days of life were characterized by very poor perfusion to essentially all body organs and tissues.

At necropsy, there were large bilateral pleural and abdominal effusions, severe centrilobular hepatic necrosis, renal tubular necrosis, focal left ventricular necrosis, and occluding thrombi in the brachiocephalic and subclavian veins and in the left internal carotid artery.

The aortic findings at necropsy are summarized partially in Figure 4.

The wall of the innominate artery aneurysm (excised at operation) was greatly thickened. The wall of the ascending aorta behind the sinuses of Valsalva was not thickened, but beginning at the sinotubular junction and extending to the origin of the celiac axis, the wall of the aorta was severely thickened (Figures 5 and 6). The lumen of the celiac axis just as it arose from the aorta was severely narrowed by the same process affecting the aorta. The wall of the abdominal aorta was normal. Histologic study of the wall of the in-

[a]Department of Internal Medicine, Division of Cardiology, and [b]Department of Pathology, [c]Baylor Heart and Vascular Institute; and [d]Departments of Radiology and [e]Cardiothoracic Surgery, Baylor University Medical Center, Dallas, Texas. Manuscript received June 16, 2009; revised manuscript received and accepted June 17, 2009.

*Corresponding author: Tel: 214-820-7911; fax: 214-820-7533.

*E-mail address:* wc.roberts@baylorhealth.edu (W.C. Roberts).

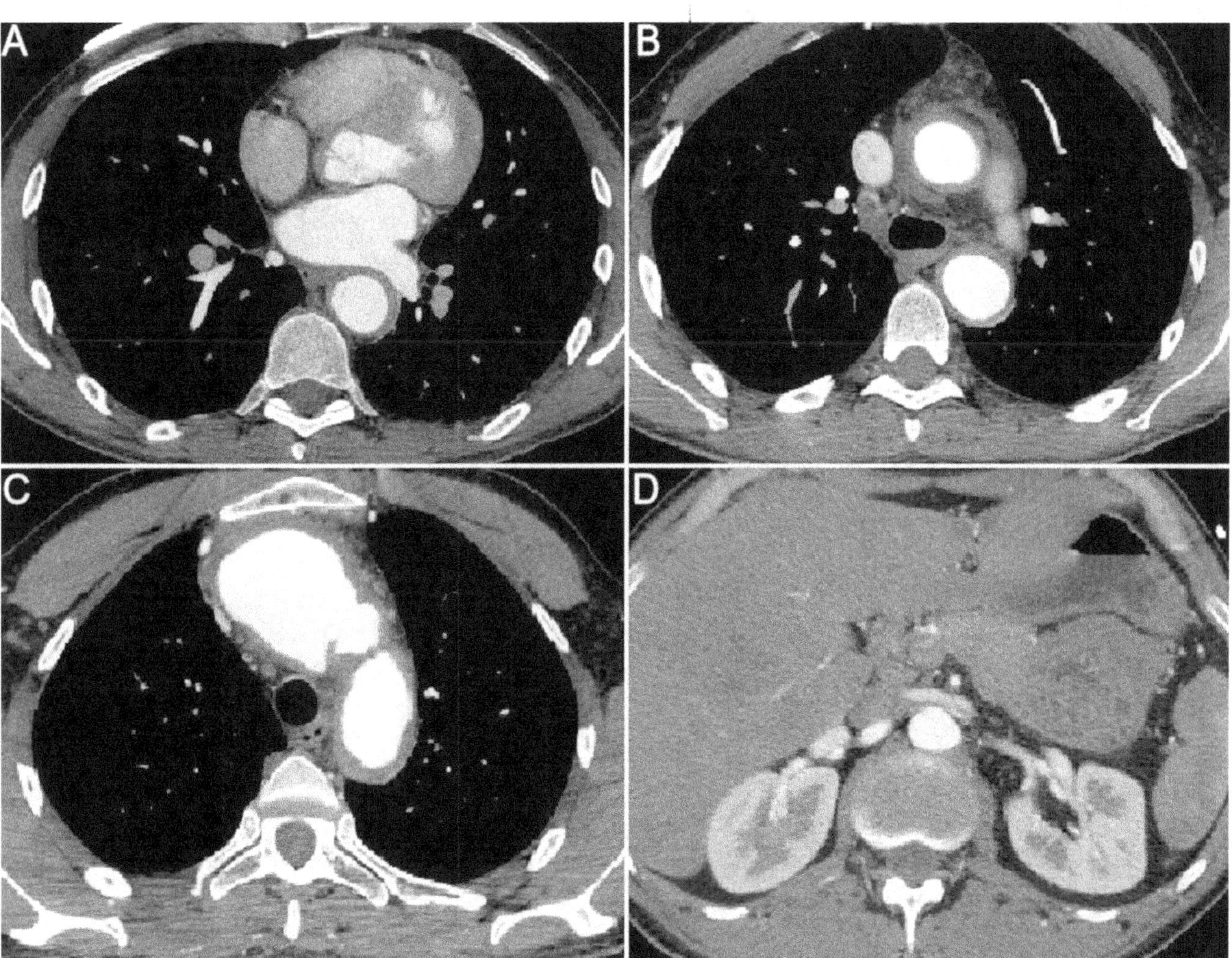

Figure 1. Computed tomographic angiographic images in the patient described. *(A)* Axial image depicting the normal appearance of the aortic root with normal wall thickness. Note also wall thickening of the descending aorta. *(B)* Axial image demonstrating severe thickening of the wall of ascending aorta with extensive inflammatory stranding in the prevascular space anterior to the ascending aorta. *(C)* Axial image of the large saccular aneurysm of the innominate artery. This image does not depict the fusiform dilatation of the more distal innominate artery. This image does not demonstrate fusiform dilatation of the distal innominate artery. from which the right subclavian and right common carotid arteries arose. *(D)* Axial demonstrating normal wall thickness of the abdominal aorta.

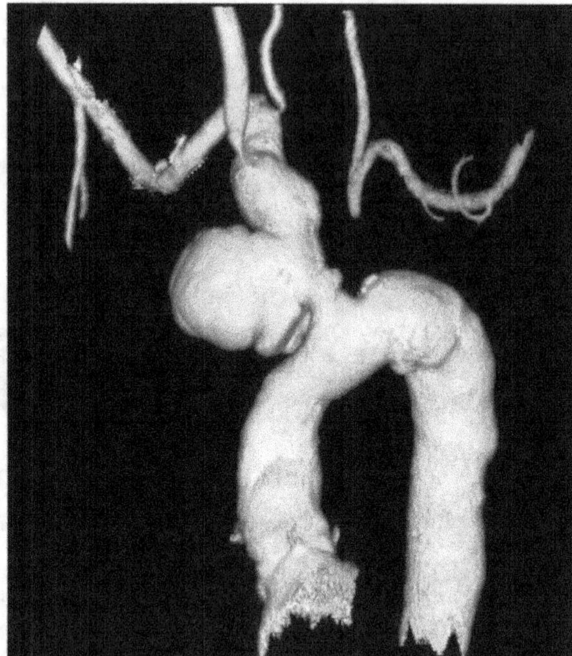

Figure 2. Computed tomographic 3-dimensional reconstruction image demonstrating the large saccular aneurysm of the proximal innominate artery, the fusiform aneurysmal dilatation of the distal innominate artery, and severe stenosis of the right common carotid artery and the origin of the right vertebral artery. This image also demonstrates complete occlusion of the left common carotid and left vertebral artery origins, with back filling of the proximal left vertebral artery. This pattern of obstruction resulted in a left-sided left subclavian steal phenomenon.

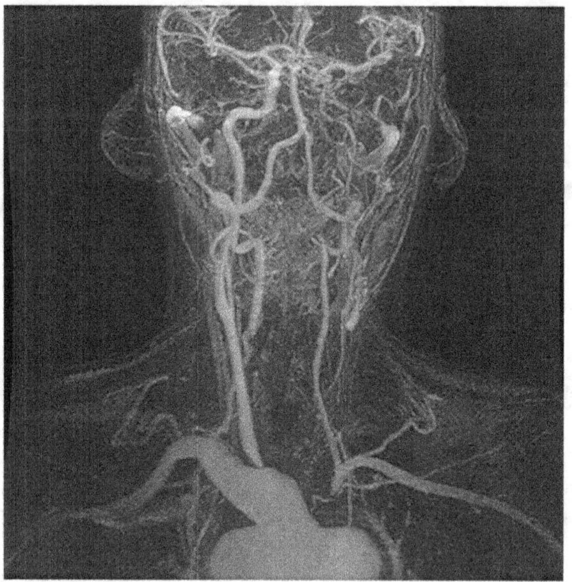

Figure 3. Maximum-intensity projection image from intracranial and extracranial gadolinium-enhanced magnetic resonance angiography demonstrating the fusiform dilatation of the distal innominate artery with severe stenosis of the right common carotid and right vertebral arteries at their origins. The left vertebral artery received backflow from the collaterals from the circle of Willis, resulting in left-sided subclavian steal. The left common carotid and left internal carotid arteries were occluded. Cerebral blood flow essentially was maintained via the right common carotid and right vertebral arteries and by perfusion to the left cerebral hemisphere via circle of Willis collaterals (anterior and posterior communicating arteries), not well visualized in this image.

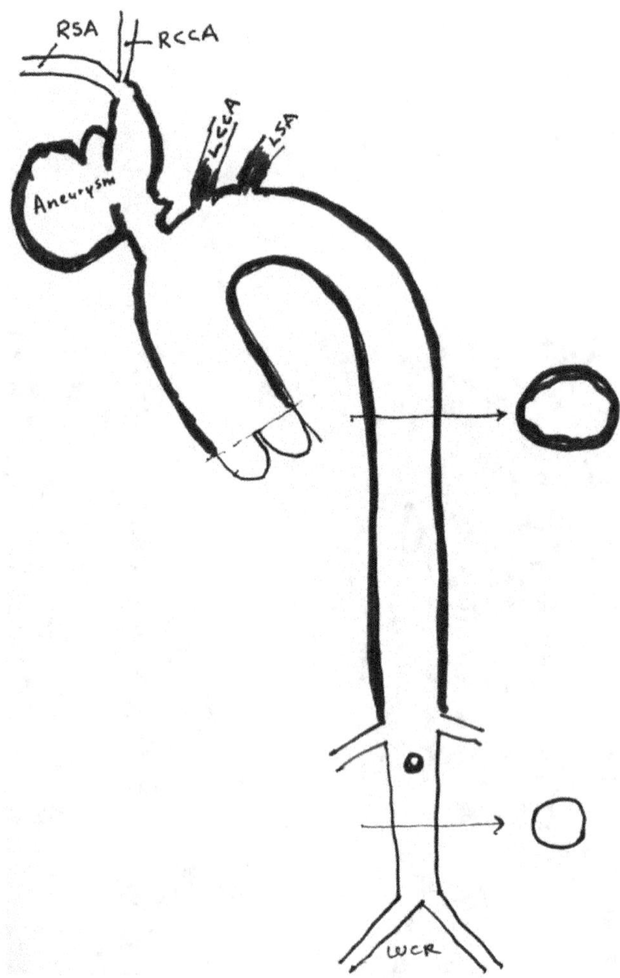


Figure 4. Diagram of aorta and aortic arch branches demonstrating the distribution of syphilitic involvement. Syphilitic involvement started at the sinotubular junction of the aorta and extended just beyond the origin of the renal arteries. The aneurysm of the innominate artery was of the saccular type, and its wall was as thick as the wall of the entire thoracic aorta distal to the sinuses of Valsalva. The origin of the right common carotid artery (RCCA) was severely narrowed, and the proximal portions of the left common carotid artery (LCCA) and left subclavian artery (LSA) were totally occluded. The celiac axis located just caudal to the origins of the renal arteries was also severely narrowed. The wall of the abdominal aorta was entirely normal, in contrast to the marked thickening of the wall of the thoracic aorta. RSA = right subclavian artery.

nominate artery aneurysm showed its wall to be similar to that of the thoracic aorta and typical of cardiovascular syphilis (Figure 7).

## Comments

The unusual features of this case are the extent of involvement of the aorta and the severe involvement of the arteries arising from the aortic arch, including a large saccular aneurysm of the innominate artery. The morphologic features of the aorta and arch arteries and celiac axis are typical of cardiovascular syphilis and confirmed by the strongly reactive serologic test for syphilis.

Aneurysm of the innominate artery has been described previously in cardiovascular syphilis. Warfield[1] described

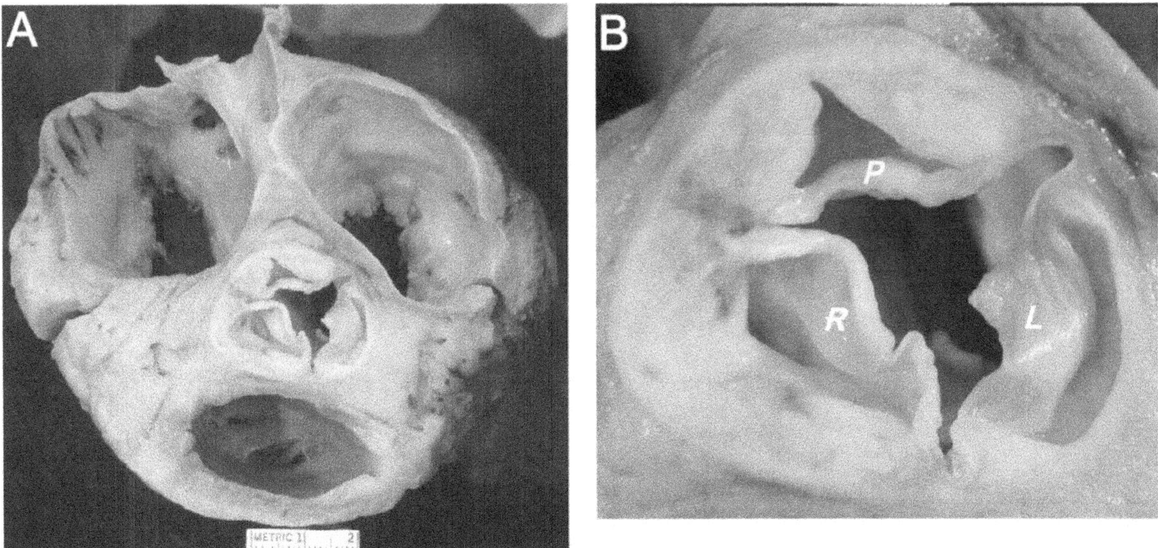

Figure 5. Heart of the patient described. *(A)* View from the cephalad direction of the right atrium, left atrium, aortic valve, and right ventricular outflow tract. *(B)* Close-up view of the aortic valve from above. The incision in the aorta is in the tubular portion just above the right (R) and posterior (P) cusps but in the sinus portion in the left (L) cusp. The sinus wall of the aorta was of normal thickness. The right coronary artery arose from the right cusp, and the wall of this aorta was of normal thickness because it was within the sinus. There was mild thickening of the margins of 2 cusps.

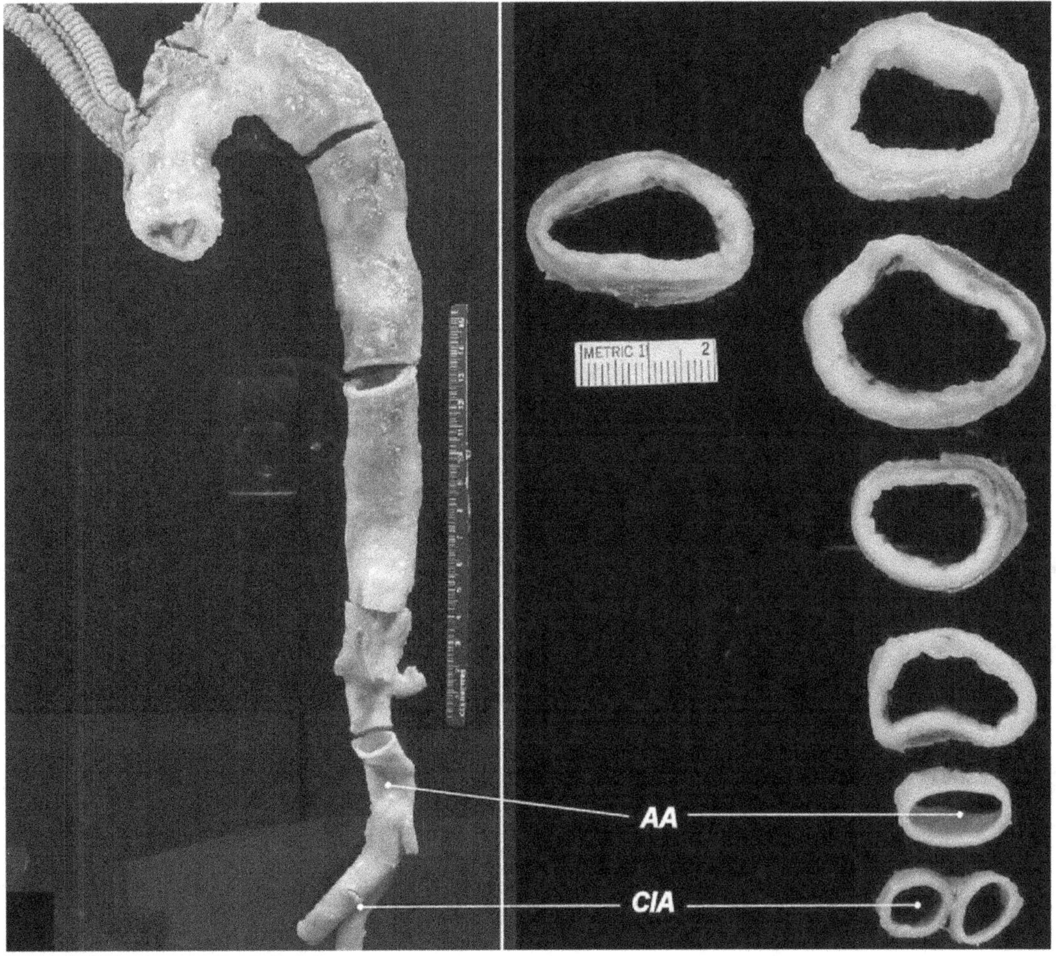



Figure 6. Tubular portion of the ascending aorta and the entire descending thoracic and abdominal aorta. The wall of the thoracic aorta was very thick, and the wall of the abdominal aorta (AA) was entirely normal. Likewise, the walls of the common iliac arteries (CIA) were entirely normal.

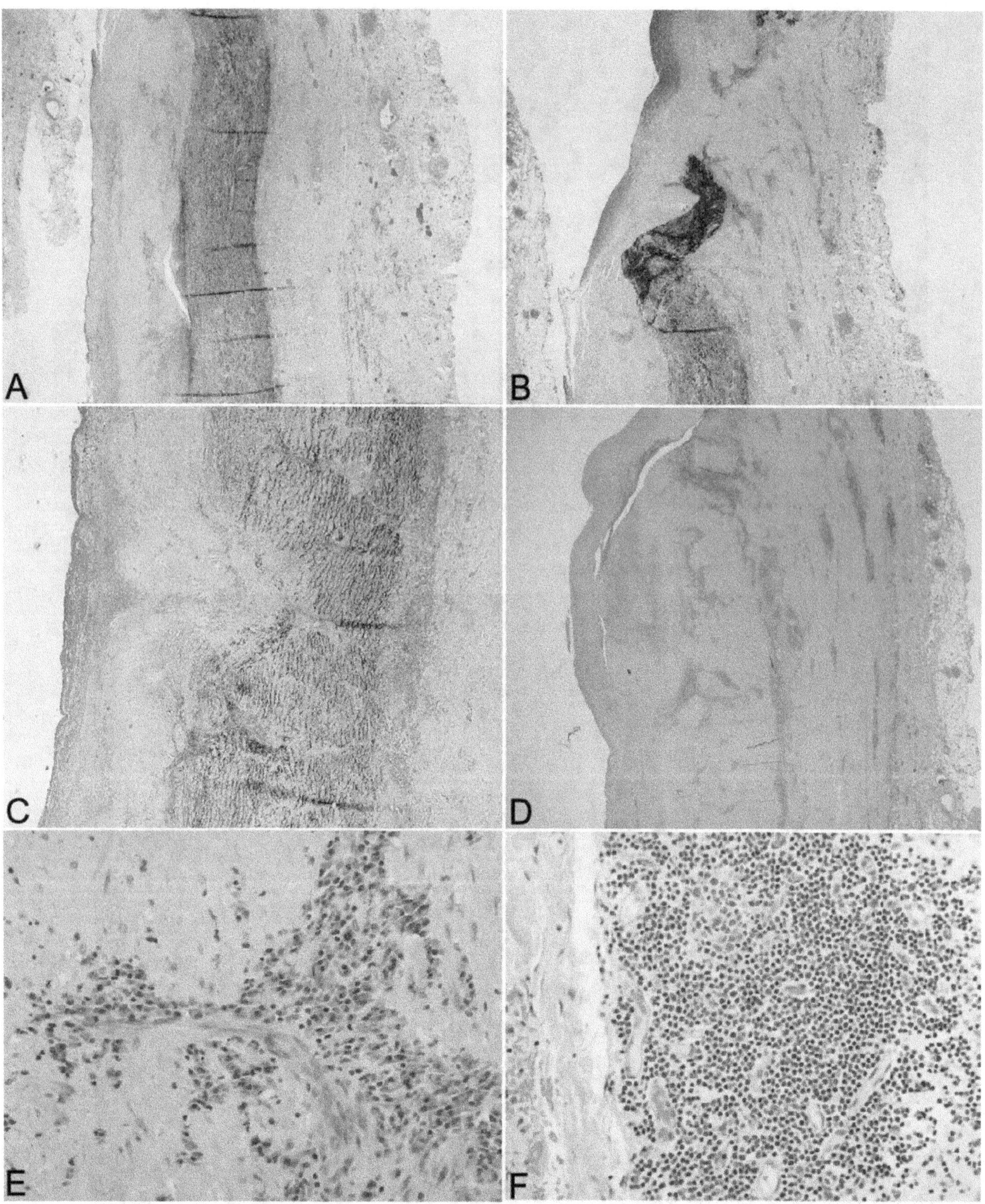

Figure 7. Histologic sections of the wall of the innominate artery aneurysm. The wall in all sections *(A to D)* was extremely thick. *(A to C)* Movat tissue stains showing marked disruption of the elastic fibers of the media, indeed a total disruption of the media in *(B)*, and marked thickening of the intima and adventitia. *(D)* Collections of inflammatory cells in both adventitia and media. *(E,F)* Close-up of the inflammatory cells, consisting of plasmacytes and lymphocytes. *(A to C)* Movat stains at 20× and hematoxylin-eosin stains at *(D)* 20× and *(E,F)* 400×.

x-ray changes in 20 patients, and the aneurysms measured 2.4 to 9.0 cm in diameter and each contained thrombus. Neither the right nor the left subclavian or internal carotid arteries were involved in the "destructive process." The patients ranged in age from 35 to 72 years. The Wassermann reaction was positive in 15 (75%). All had severe involvement of the thoracic aorta. Twelve were studied at necropsy. Gay and Walker[2] described x-ray features of 18 patients, all men, aged 35 to 63 years, with innominate artery aneurysms. Fourteen (78%) had positive serologic results for syphilis, and 7 (39%) had histories of chancres. Tadavarthy et al[3] reported 4 patients with syphilis involving the thoracic aorta, including a saccular aneurysm of the innominate artery. All 4 patients had positive Venereal Disease Research Laboratory test results for syphilis. Goei et al[4] described a 66-year-old man with an aneurysm of the innominate artery, a very dilated ascending aorta, and a history of having been treated for syphilis 20 years earlier.

Characteristically in cardiovascular syphilis, the wall of the aorta behind the sinuses of Valsalva is spared, and the process begins immediately at the sinotubular junction. Distal to the sinotubular junction, every square millimeter of the aorta was affected until just past the origin of the celiac axis, and from that point distally, the aorta was normal.


1. Warfield CH. Roentgen diagnosis of aneurysms of the innominate artery. *AJR Am J Roentgenol* 1935;33:350–358.
2. Gay BB Jr, Walker FJ. Aneurysm of the innominate artery: review of clinical and radiologic findings in 18 cases. *Radiology* 1953;60:804–813.
3. Tadavarthy SM, Castaneda-Zuniga WR, Klugman J, Shachar JB, Amplatz K. Syphilitic aneurysms of the innominate artery. *Radiology* 1981;139:31–34.
4. Goei R, Tjwa MK, Snoep G. Luetic aneurysm of the innominate artery mimicking a mass in the right side of the anterior mediastinum: MR appearance. *AJR Am J Roentgenol* 1992;159:1343.

# Electrocardiographic Total 12-Lead QRS Voltage in Patients Having Operative Resection of Syphilitic Aortic Aneurysm

William C. Roberts, MD[a,b,c,*], Clay M. Barbin, MD[a], Matthew R. Weissenborn, MD[d], and Jong M. Ko, BA[c]

Electrocardiographic voltage has been used to determine the presence of left ventricular hypertrophy for about 70 years. Varying electrocardiographic criteria have been applied. We have found total 12-lead QRS voltage to be most useful in this regard. We measured total 12-lead QRS voltage in 24 patients in whom an ascending aortic aneurysm was resected and histologic study of its wall was classic of syphilitic aortitis. In these 24 patients total 12-lead QRS voltage ranged from 57 to 161 mm, averaging 120 ± 32 in the 11 men and 106 ± 24 mm in the 13 women. If normal 12-lead QRS voltage in adults is considered to be >175 mm not a single one of the 24 patients had normal voltage. Indeed, most were in the low normal area. Thus, this study provides some evidence via this indirect means that the heart itself is infrequently involved by syphilitic aortitis which produces an ascending aortic aneurysm of sufficient size to warrant resection.   © 2015 Elsevier Inc. All rights reserved. (Am J Cardiol 2015;116:973−976)

During the past 30 years we have compared electrocardiographic total 12-lead QRS voltage to heart weight at necropsy or after cardiac transplantation in 11 different cardiac conditions.[1–11] These studies were summarized in a recent review, which also demonstrated that total 12-lead QRS voltage was the best electrocardiographic indicator of increased cardiac mass.[12] Our necropsy studies in patients with syphilitic aortitis have indicated that, with few exceptions, the heart is of normal size.[13] The present study examines total 12-lead QRS voltage in 24 patients who underwent operative resection of a thoracic syphilitic aneurysm to determine if any had evidence of increased cardiac mass using this indirect criterion.

## Methods

From 2010 through 2014, twenty-four patients have had resection of a syphilitic aneurysm involving the ascending aorta at Baylor University Medical Center at Dallas, and each had an immediate preoperative electrocardiogram available for examination. The QRS voltage (from the peak of the R wave to the nadir of either the Q or the S wave, whichever was deeper [Figure 1]) was measured in each of the 12 leads in each of the 24 patients and certain other clinical features also were collected.

Departments of [a]Internal Medicine, [b]Pathology, and [d]Radiology, Baylor University Medical Center, Dallas, Texas; and [c]Baylor Heart and Vascular Institute, Baylor University Medical Center, Dallas, Texas. Manuscript received June 3, 2015; revised manuscript received and accepted June 16, 2015.

The study was funded by the Baylor Health Care Foundation.

See page 975 for disclosure information.

*Corresponding author: Tel: (214) 820-7911; fax: (214) 820-7533.

*E-mail address:* wc.roberts@baylorhealth.edu (W.C. Roberts).

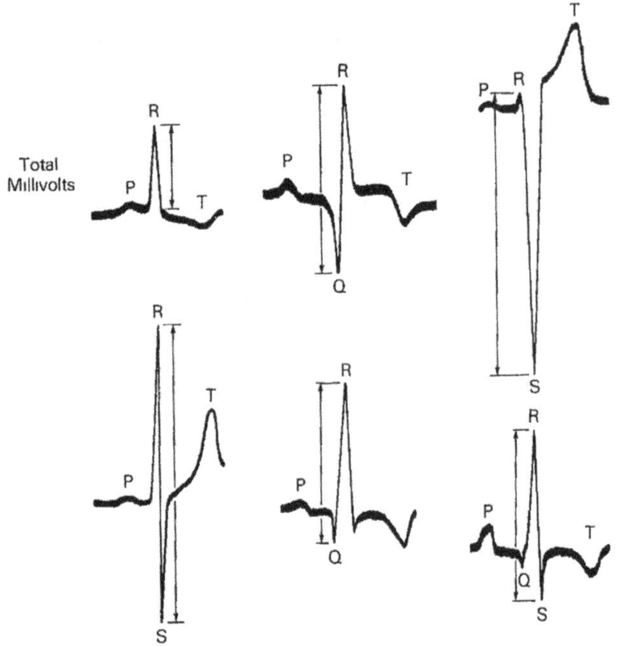


Figure 1. Various QRS complexes showing how each was measured. (Reproduced with permission: Siegel RJ, Roberts WC. *Am Heart J* 1982;103:210-221.[1]).

## Results

Pertinent findings in each of the 24 patients are summarized in Table 1. Total 12-lead QRS voltage (measured with normal [10 mm] standardization [10 mm = 1 mV]) in the 11 men (mean age 61 ± 17 years) ranged from 57 to 161 mm (mean 120 ± 32), and in the 13 women (mean age 71 ± 9 years), from 64 to 146 mm (mean 106 ± 24). All but one of the 24 patients had a history of systemic

Table 1
Certain clinical and electrocardiographic features of cases of syphilitic aortitis at Baylor University Medical Center from January 1. 2009 to December 31. 2014

| # | Age (years) | RACE | BMI (Kg/m2) | QRS Amplitude in Each Electrocardiographic lead | | | | | | | | | | | | | | TC (mg/dl) | LDL (mg/dl) | Coronary Angiography Done | No. of CA Narrrowed | CT Asc Aorta An Diameter (cm) | Cardiac Catheterization | | | | AVR |
|---|---|---|---|---|---|---|---|---|---|---|---|---|---|---|---|---|---|---|---|---|---|---|---|---|---|---|---|
| | | | | I | II | III | aVR | aVL | aVF | V1 | V2 | V3 | V4 | V5 | V6 | QRSTOTAL | BBB | | | | | | LV (s/d) (mmHg) | SA (s/d) (mmHg) | EF (%) | CI (L/min/m$^2$) | |
| **MEN** | | | | | | | | | | | | | | | | | | | | | | | | | | | |
| 1 | 33 | W | 24.7 | 11 | 9 | 5 | 9 | 9 | 5 | 12 | 17 | 12 | 22 | 23 | 17 | 151 | 0 | 184 | 96 | + | 0 | | 133/26 | 133/73 | 60 | 3.1 | + |
| 2 | 45 | B | 23 | 3 | 12 | 10 | 6 | 5 | 11 | 11 | 10 | 21 | 25 | 17 | 11 | 142 | 0 | - | - | 0 | - | 8.2 | - | 180/100 (I) | 55 (E) | - | 0 |
| 3 | 48 | B | 27.9 | 8 | 10 | 6 | 9 | 3 | 9 | 13 | 16 | 9 | 21 | 21 | 15 | 140 | 0 | 218 | 147 | 0 | - | 6.2 | - | 121/77 (I) | 60 (E) | - | 0 |
| 4 | 51 | W | 28.1 | 9 | 5 | 5 | 7 | 7 | 4 | 12 | 11 | 20 | 34 | 29 | 18 | 161 | 0 | 151 | 97 | + | 0 | 7.4 | 144/22 | 131/60 | 35 | 2.4 | 0 |
| 5 | 59 | A | 28.4 | 7 | 7 | 5 | 6 | 5 | 4 | 7 | 12 | 12 | 12 | 14 | 16 | 152 | 0 | 186 | 118 | 0 | - | 4.7 | - | 120/80 (I) | 74 (E) | - | 0 |
| 6 | 59 | B | 34.4 | 5 | 7 | 3 | 5 | 2 | 4 | 2 | 6 | 18 | 25 | 23 | 18 | 118 | 0 | - | - | 0 | - | AD | - | 111/65 (I) | 65 (E) | - | + |
| 7 | 60 | W | 28.9 | 8 | 2 | 7 | 5 | 8 | 4 | 5 | 15 | 17 | 18 | 11 | 9 | 109 | 0 | 225 | 156 | + | 0 | - | 145/23 | 14/85(I) | 63 | 1.6 | 0 |
| 8 | 70 | W | 37.7 | 9 | 3 | 8 | 6 | 9 | 3 | 7 | 9 | 11 | 12 | 12 | 13 | 102 | 0 | 136 | 88 | + | 3(CABG)* | 6.7 | 173/33 | 170/33 | 45 | - | 0 |
| 9 | 80 | W | 28 | 6 | 4 | 6 | 3 | 6 | 5 | 7 | 6 | 15 | 21 | 18 | 11 | 108 | +R | 108 | 49 | + | 1 (CABG) | 5.7 | 129/9 | 130/59 | 55 | 3.4 | 0 |
| 10 | 83 | W | 24.4 | 6 | 19 | 5 | 5 | 6 | 2 | 5 | 5 | 10 | 11 | 3 | 9 | 86 | 0 | 128 | 81 | + | 2 (CABG)* | - | 133/10 | 132/59 | 35 | 3.2 | + |
| 11 | 84 | W | 26.5 | 5 | 5 | 4 | 4 | 4 | 3 | 6 | 4 | 4 | 5 | 7 | 6 | 57 | 0 | 126 | 79 | + | 1 (CABG) | - | 121/19 | 103/63 | 45 | - | + |
| | 33-84 | | 23-37.7 | | | | | | | | | | | | | 57-161 | | | | | | | | | | | |
| | (61±17) | | (28.4±4.3) | | | | | | | | | | | | | (120±32) | | | | | | | | | | | |
| **WOMEN** | | | | | | | | | | | | | | | | | | | | | | | | | | | |
| 1 | 58 | B | 31.7 | 4 | 7 | 9 | 5 | 6 | 8 | 4 | 11 | 10 | 14 | 15 | 10 | 103 | 0 | 184 | 110 | + | 0 | 5.1 | 126/3 | 125/80 | 60 | - | 0 |
| 2 | 59 | W | 28.9 | 19 | 15 | 4 | 14 | 9 | 6 | 11 | 9 | 13 | 16 | 16 | 14 | 146 | 0 | 190 | 110 | + | 0 | 6.6 | - | 156/83 | 60 (E) | - | + |
| 3 | 62 | W | 45.6 | 8 | 6 | 4 | 7 | 5 | 4 | 14 | 17 | 25 | 9 | 11 | 12 | 122 | 0 | 199 | 141 | + | 0 | 5.1 | 152/26 | 153/45 | 50 | 2.7 | + |
| 4 | 65 | W | 46.5 | 6 | 4 | 3 | 5 | 4 | 2 | 3 | 12 | 8 | 11 | 12 | 8 | 78 | 0 | 129 | 65 | + | 0 | 6.4 | 114/16 | 117/67 | 65 (E) | - | 0 |
| 5 | 65 | W | 28.9 | 7 | 4 | 6 | 6 | 7 | 3 | 7 | 12 | 17 | 19 | 20 | 14 | 122 | 0 | 129 | 65 | 0 | - | 6 | 153/13 | 154/83 | 70 | - | 0 |
| 6 | 67 | W | 26.2 | 12 | 9 | 8 | 10 | 9 | 6 | 12 | 16 | 13 | 11 | 10 | 9 | 125 | 0 | 86 | 47 | + | 0 | - | 124/4 | 125/83 | 60 | 2.9 | 0 |
| 7 | 69 | W | 15.8 | 2 | 10 | 8 | 6 | 4 | 10 | 4 | 4 | 5 | 10 | 14 | 23 | 100 | 0 | 158 | 84 | + | 2 | 5.6 | 101/3 | 100/60 | 55 | - | 0 |
| 8 | 70 | W | 21.6 | 5 | 6 | 4 | 6 | 3 | 4 | 4 | 10 | 15 | 18 | 25 | 14 | 114 | 0 | 142 | 69 | + | 0 | 5.4 | - | 156/57 | 63 (E) | - | 0 |
| 9 | 78 | B | 25.1 | 9 | 8 | 8 | 7 | 7 | 6 | 10 | 6 | 9 | 13 | 15 | 12 | 111 | 0 | 167 | 112 | + | 1 (CABG)* | - | - | 134/88 (I) | - | - | +† |
| 10 | 79 | W | 24.8 | 5 | 7 | 4 | 6 | 3 | 5 | 9 | 7 | 5 | 4 | 4 | 11 | 70 | 0 | - | - | + | 3 | 5.2 | - | 143/57 (I) | 60 (E) | - | + |
| 11 | 80 | W | 28.6 | 4 | 11 | 12 | 4 | 6 | 10 | 6 | 9 | 7 | 9 | 10 | 11 | 99 | 0 | - | - | + | 0 | 5.7 | 144/27 | 140/54 | 60 | 3.1 | 0 |
| 12 | 83 | W | 22.3 | 5 | 4 | 3 | 4 | 4 | 3 | 4 | 11 | 3 | 10 | 8 | 5 | 64 | 0 | - | - | + | 0 | - | 124/13 | 123/58 | 60 | 3.7 | 0 |
| 13 | 83 | W | 18.6 | 8 | 6 | 4 | 6 | 5 | 6 | 10 | 10 | 14 | 23 | 17 | 11 | 120 | +R | 79 | 39 | + | 0 | - | 182/18 | 179/54 | 55 | 2.8 | + |
| | 58-83 | | 15.8-46.5 | | | | | | | | | | | | | 64-146 | | | | | | | | | | | |
| | (71±9) | | (28.0±9.1) | | | | | | | | | | | | | (106±24) | | | | | | | | | | | |

AVR = aortic valve replacement; B = black; BBB = bundle branch block; BMI = body mass index; Cas = coronary arteries; CABG = coronary artery bypass grafting; CI = cardiac index; CT = computed tomographic; E = echo; EF = ejection fraction; I = indirect; LDL = low-density lipoprotein cholesterol; LV = left ventricle; R = right; SA = systemic artery; s/d = peak systole/end diastole; TC = total cholesterol; W = white; - = not available.

* CABG was done in the past.

† Aortic repair was due to aortic aneurysm; AVR was due to aortic regurgitation, and CABG were performed 11 years earlier.

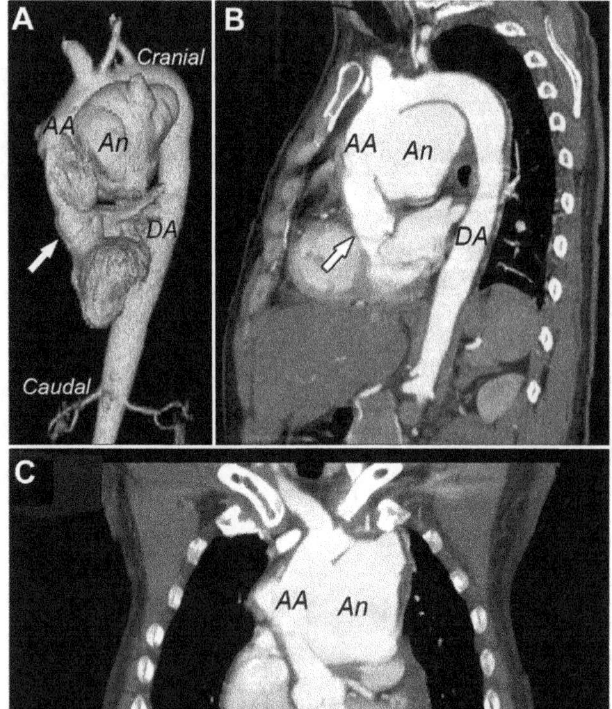

Figure 2. Table 1, Men, Patient #2. *(A)* Volume rendered 3-Dimensional reconstruction, *(B)* contrast enhanced sagittal maximum intensity projection, and *(C)* contrast enhanced coronal CT images reveal a large, wide-necked multilobulated saccular aneurysm (An) arising from the posterolateral aspect of the ascending aorta (AA) and extending posteriorly. Note the aortic sinus is unaffected *(white arrows)*. DA = descending aorta; LV = left ventricle.

hypertension. Echocardiograms, available for review in 4 of the 24 patients, disclosed left ventricular wall thicknesses $\leq 1.2$ cm in all 4 patients, left ventricular ejection fractions $\geq 55\%$ in all 4, aortic regurgitation in 4 (all minimal or mild), and a dilated left ventricular cavity in none. Computed tomographic imaging preoperatively, data available in 15 of the 24 patients, showed the maximal diameter of the ascending aorta to range from 4.7 to 8.2 cm (mean 6.5 in 6 men and 5.7 in 9 women). The body mass index (Kg/m$^2$) ranged from 23 to 38 (mean 28 $\pm$ 4) in the 11 men, and from 15 to 47 (mean 28 $\pm$ 9) in the 13 women. Data from coronary angiography, available in 18 patients, disclosed narrowing of 1 or more major coronary arteries in 6 (33%) patients and 4 of the 6 underwent coronary artery bypass grafting. Serum total cholesterol levels (15 patients) ranged from 79 to 225 mg/dl (mean 163) and was >200 mg/dl in only 3 patients; low-density lipoprotein cholesterol ranged from 39 to 164 mg/dl (mean 100) and was >100 mg/dl in 6 of the 15 patients.

Left ventricular data from cardiac catheterization were available in 15 patients (Table 1). The peak left ventricular systolic pressure ranged from 102 to 182 mm Hg (average 135) and simultaneous systemic arterial pressure ranged from 100 to 182 mm Hg (average 132). Left ventricular angiography disclosed the left ventricular cavity to be dilated in only 2 (13%) of the 15 patients. The left ventricular ejection fractions ranged from 35 to 70% (mean 56), and was below 50% in only 2 patients. The cardiac indexes ranged from 1.6 to 3.7 ml/minute/m$^2$ (mean 2.9) and was <2.5 in 2 of 10 patients where the data was recorded.

The ascending aorta was resected in all 24 patients (Figure 2) and histologic examination in each showed typical findings of syphilitic aortitis. Additionally, the aortic valve was replaced in 7 of the 24 patients.

## Comments

This study found, among patients having resection of an aneurysm of the ascending aorta with histologic features of the aneurysmal wall typical of syphilis,[13] that the total 12-lead QRS voltage was normal (<175 mm) in all 24 patients, providing evidence that the cardiac mass is usually normal in patients with syphilitic aortitis. Not only was the total 12-lead QRS voltage normal in the 24 patients but it was in the low-normal range (mean 112 mm) similar to that in patients with massive cardiac adiposity (mean 120 mm); cardiac amyloidosis (mean 104 mm), and the carcinoid syndrome (mean 105 mm).[12] In contrast, total 12-lead QRS voltage in patients with aortic stenosis averaged 273 mm; those with pure aortic regurgitation (no element of aortic stenosis), 272 mm; mitral regurgitation, 220 mm; hypertrophic cardiomyopathy, 195 mm, and idiopathic dilated cardiomyopathy, 153 mm.[12]

From the electrocardiographic, echocardiographic, and morphologic aspects syphilis does not affect the heart or if so only in a secondary manner. Syphilis when involving the vascular system is a disease of the thoracic aorta and the arch arteries. When aortic regurgitation does occur, it is the result of the disease in the aorta and the process does not affect, except in a secondary manner, the aortic valve cusps. When a coronary ostium is narrowed in syphilis it is the result of the aortitis, not direct involvement of the coronary artery itself. Thus, the phrase "cardiovascular syphilis" might best be dropped and replaced by "syphilitic aortitis" or "vascular syphilis."

A positive feature of the present study is the fact that total 12-lead QRS voltage has not been described previously in patients with thoracic aneurysm. Limitations include little echocardiographic data and the absence of cardiac weights.

## Disclosures

The authors have no conflicts of interest to disclose.


1. Siegel RJ, Roberts WC. Electrocardiographic observations in severe aortic valve stenosis: correlative necropsy study to clinical, hemodynamic, and ECG variables demonstrating relation of 12-lead QRS amplitude to peak systolic transaortic pressure gradient. *Am Heart J* 1982;103:210–221.
2. Roberts WC, Podolak MJ. The king of hearts: analysis of 23 patients with hearts weighing 1000 grams or more. *Am J Cardiol* 1985;55:485–494.
3. Roberts WC, Day PJ. Electrocardiographic observations in clinically isolated, pure, chronic, severe aortic regurgitation: analysis of 30 necropsy patients aged 19 to 65 years. *Am J Cardiol* 1985;55:432–438.

4. Glick BN, Roberts WC. Usefulness of total 12-lead QRS voltage in diagnosing left ventricular hypertrophy in clinically isolated, pure, chronic, severe mitral regurgitation. *Am J Cardiol* 1992;70:1088–1092.

5. Dollar AL, Roberts WC. Usefulness of total 12-lead QRS voltage compared with other criteria for determining left ventricular hypertrophy in hypertrophic cardiomyopathy: analysis of 57 patients studied at necropsy. *Am J Med* 1989;87:377–381.

6. Shirani J, Maron BJ, Cannon RO III, Shahin S, Roberts WC. Clinicopathologic features of hypertrophic cardiomyopathy managed by cardiac transplantation. *Am J Cardiol* 1993;72:434–440.

7. Roberts WC, Siegel RJ, McManus BM. Idiopathic dilated cardiomyopathy: analysis of 152 necropsy patients. *Am J Cardiol* 1987;60:1340–1355.

8. Shirani J, Roberts WC. Clinical electrocardiographic and morphologic features of massive fatty deposits ("lipomatous hypertrophy") in the atrial septum. *J Am Coll Cardiol* 1993;22:226–238.

9. Ross EM, Roberts WC. The carcinoid syndrome: comparison of 21 necropsy subjects with carcinoid heart disease to 15 necropsy subjects without carcinoid heart disease. *Am J Med* 1985;79:339–354.

10. Roberts WC, Waller BF. Cardiac amyloidosis causing cardiac dysfunction: analysis of 54 necropsy patients. *Am J Cardiol* 1983;52:137–146.

11. Shirani J, Berezowski K, Roberts WC. Quantitative measurement of normal and excessive (cor adiposum) subepicardial adipose tissue, its clinical significance, and its effect on electrocardiographic QRS voltage. *Am J Cardiol* 1995;76:414–418.

12. Roberts WC, Filardo G, Ko JM, Siegel RJ, Dollar AL, Ross EM, Shirani J. Comparison of total 12-lead QRS voltage in a variety of cardiac conditions and its usefulness in predicting increased cardiac mass. *Am J Cardiol* 2013;112:904–909.

13. Roberts WC, Ko JM, Vowels TJ. Natural history of syphilitic aortitis. *Am J Cardiol* 2009;104:1578–1587.

# Syphilis as a Cause of Thoracic Aortic Aneurysm

William C. Roberts, MD[a,b,c,*], Clay M. Barbin, MD[a], Matthew R. Weissenborn, MD[d], Jong M. Ko, BA[c], and A. Carl Henry, MD[e]

In 2009, we described morphologic findings in 22 patients having resection of an ascending aortic aneurysm in the previous 11 years at the Baylor University Medical Center, and histologic examination of the aneurysmal wall disclosed classic findings of syphilitic aortitis. The major purpose of that extensively illustrated report was to describe the characteristic gross features of the aneurysm such that syphilitic aortitis might be better recognized at operation and appropriate antibiotics administered postoperatively. The aim of the present study was to emphasize that syphilis remains a major cause of ascending aortic aneurysm. From January 1, 2009, to December 31, 2014, we studied additional 23 patients who had resection of an ascending aortic aneurysm that again histologically had classic features of syphilitic aortitis. All 23 patients were found to have syphilitic aortitis grossly and histologically. The aneurysm involved the ascending portion of aorta in all 23, the arch portion in 12, and the descending thoracic portion in 10. In conclusion, syphilis has far from disappeared. It remains a major cause of ascending aortic aneurysm. © 2015 Elsevier Inc. All rights reserved. (Am J Cardiol 2015;116:1298−1303)

In 2009, we described finding in 22 patients who underwent operative resection of an ascending aortic aneurysm at the Baylor University Medical Center (BUMC) from 1998 to 2008, and histologic examination of the aneurysmal wall was typical of syphilitic aortitis.[1] The emphasis of that report was the describing of the morphologic features of syphilitic aortitis so that the condition could be more readily diagnosed at operation and also to emphasize that syphilis as a cause of thoracic aortic aneurysm had not disappeared. The present study was prompted by studying an additional 23 patients who underwent resection of an ascending aortic aneurysm caused by syphilitic aortitis at the same institution during the subsequent 6 years, again to emphasize that this condition has far from disappeared.

## Methods

Since March 1993, all operatively excised specimens excised by cardiovascular surgeons at the BUMC have been described grossly and histologically by WCR and photographed mainly by JMK, and since 2003, the clinical records were available online. From January 1, 2009, to December 31, 2014, 23 patients were found to have diffuse panaortitis of the tubular portion of ascending aorta. The diffuseness of the involvement of the ascending aorta was determined by gross examination and the panaortitis by histologic examination. Takayasu's arteritis was ruled out by the absence of giant cells in any layer of the aneurysmal wall.[2,3] Ankylosing spondylitis was ruled out by the absence of arthritic disease, by the minimal involvement of the tubular portion of ascending aorta, by extension of the process into the walls of the sinus portion of aorta and onto the bases of the aortic valve cusps, and by the extension of the process onto the anterior mitral leaflet and into the membranous ventricular septum.[4,5]

All 23 patients at operation were stated to have 3-cuspid aortic valves that were free of calcific deposits. The free margins, mainly their central portions, were described as being mildly thickened in some patients. The sinus portion of aorta was not dilated or described as being abnormal.

A positive or reactive serologic test for syphilis (STS) was not considered a criterion for inclusion in the present study because the test was never done in most patients, or, if performed, the results were unavailable.

## Results

Pertinent findings in each of the 23 patients are listed in Table 1. The 11 men ranged in age from 33 to 84 years (mean 61), and the 12 women from 58 to 83 years (mean 70). Eighteen were white; 4, black; and 1, Asian. The body mass index ranged from 16 to 47 kg/m$^2$ (mean 28); it was >25 in 15 (65%).

The aneurysm involved the ascending portion of aorta in all 23 patients, the arch portion in 12, and the descending thoracic portion in 10. In all patients, the aneurysm was fusiform, that is, the entire aortic wall was part of the aneurysmal wall. Additionally, at least 5 patients had saccular aneurysms projecting from the fusiform

Departments of [a]Internal Medicine, [b]Pathology, [d]Radiology, [e]Cardiothoracic Surgery, and [c]The Baylor Heart and Vascular Institute, Baylor University Medical Center, Dallas, Texas. Manuscript received June 30, 2015; revised manuscript received and accepted July 3, 2015.

The study was funded by the Baylor Health Care System Foundation, 3600 Gaston Avenue, Barnett Tower, Suite 100 Dallas, TX 75246.

See page 1303 for disclosure information.

*Corresponding author: Tel: (214) 820-7911; fax: (214) 820-7533.

*E-mail address:* wc.roberts@baylorhealth.edu (W.C. Roberts).

Table 1
Surgical cases of syphilitic aortitis at Baylor University Medical Center from January 1, 2009 to December 31, 2014

| Patient | Age (years) | Race | BMI (Kg/m$^2$) | Pressures (mmHg) (s/d) | | Aneurysm | | | | | AVR | Weight of AV (g) | STS | Result | CABG |
|---|---|---|---|---|---|---|---|---|---|---|---|---|---|---|---|
| | | | | | | Location | | | Type | | | | | | |
| | | | | LV | SA | Asc | Arch | DT | Saccular | Fusiform | | | | | |
| **MEN** | | | | | | | | | | | | | | | |
| 1 | 33 | W | 24.7 | 118/27 | 132/72 | + | 0 | 0 | 0 | + | + | 0.47 | — | — | 0 |
| 2 | 45 | B | 23.0 | — | 180/100 | + | 0 | 0 | + | + | 0 | — | + | Ab, RPR 1:128 | 0 |
| 3 | 48 | B | 27.9 | — | 106/65 | + | + | 0 | + | + | 0 | — | — | — | 0 |
| 4 | 51 | W | 28.1 | 148/20 | 131/60 | + | 0 | 0 | 0 | + | 0 | — | 0 | — | 0 |
| 5 | 59 | A | 28.4 | — | 170/80 | + | + | + | + | + | 0 | — | 0 | — | 0 |
| 6 | 59 | B | 34.4 | — | 120/70 | + | + | 0 | 0 | + | + | 0.83 | 0 | — | 0 |
| 7 | 60 | W | 28.9 | 120/7 | 140/90 | + | + | 0 | 0 | + | 0 | — | 0 | — | 0 |
| 8 | 70 | W | 37.7 | 190/40 | 190/90 | + | + | + | 0 | + | 0 | — | 0 | — | + |
| 9 | 80 | W | 28.0 | 123/5 | 145/85 | + | + | + | 0 | + | 0 | — | 0 | — | + |
| 10 | 83 | W | 24.4 | 130/10 | 150/80 | + | 0 | 0 | 0 | + | + | 0.91 | 0 | — | + |
| 11 | 84 | W | 26.5 | 120/20 | 120/70 | + | + | + | 0 | + | + | 0.86 | 0 | — | + |
| | 33-84 (61±17) | | 23.0-37.7 (28.4±4.3) | | | | | | | | | | | | |
| **WOMEN** | | | | | | | | | | | | | | | |
| 1 | 58 | B | 31.7 | 126/30 | 140/90 | + | 0 | 0 | 0 | + | 0 | — | 0 | — | 0 |
| 2 | 59 | W | 28.9 | 0 | 160/90 | + | + | + | 0 | + | 0 | — | 0 | — | 0 |
| 3 | 62 | W | 45.6 | 155/25 | 170/65 | + | 0 | + | + | + | + | 0.78 | + | NR (Ab) | 0 |
| 4 | 65 | W | 46.5 | 114/16 | 120/65 | + | 0 | + | 0 | + | 0 | — | 0 | — | 0 |
| 5 | 65 | W | 28.9 | 142/10 | 130/75 | + | + | + | 0 | + | 0 | — | 0 | — | 0 |
| 6 | 67 | W | 26.2 | 124/4 | 135/60 | + | 0 | 0 | 0 | + | 0 | — | + | NR (Ab) | 0 |
| 7 | 69 | W | 15.8 | 101/3 | 100/60 | + | 0 | + | 0 | + | 0 | — | 0 | — | + |
| 8 | 70 | W | 21.6 | — | 170/80 | + | 0 | 0 | 0 | + | 0 | — | + | NR (RPR) | 0 |
| 9 | 79 | W | 24.8 | — | 140/55 | + | + | + | + | + | 0 | — | 0 | — | + |
| 10 | 80 | W | 28.6 | 145/30 | 145/60 | + | 0 | 0 | 0 | + | 0 | — | + | NR (RPR) | 0 |
| 11 | 83 | W | 18.6 | 175/20 | 175/70 | + | 0 | 0 | 0 | + | + | 0.55 | 0 | — | 0 |
| 12 | 83 | W | 22.3 | 120/10 | 120/40 | + | 0 | 0 | 0 | + | 0 | — | 0 | — | 0 |
| | 58-83 (70±9) | | 15.8-46.5 (28.3±9.5) | | | | | | | | | | | | |

A = Asian; Ab = antibody; Asc = ascending; AV = aortic valve; AVR = aortic valve replacement; B = black; BMI = body mass index; CABG = coronary artery bypass grafting; DT = descending thoracic; LV = left ventricle; NR = non-reactive; RPR = rapid plasma reagin; SA = systemic artery; STS = serologic test for syphilis; W = white; — = not available.

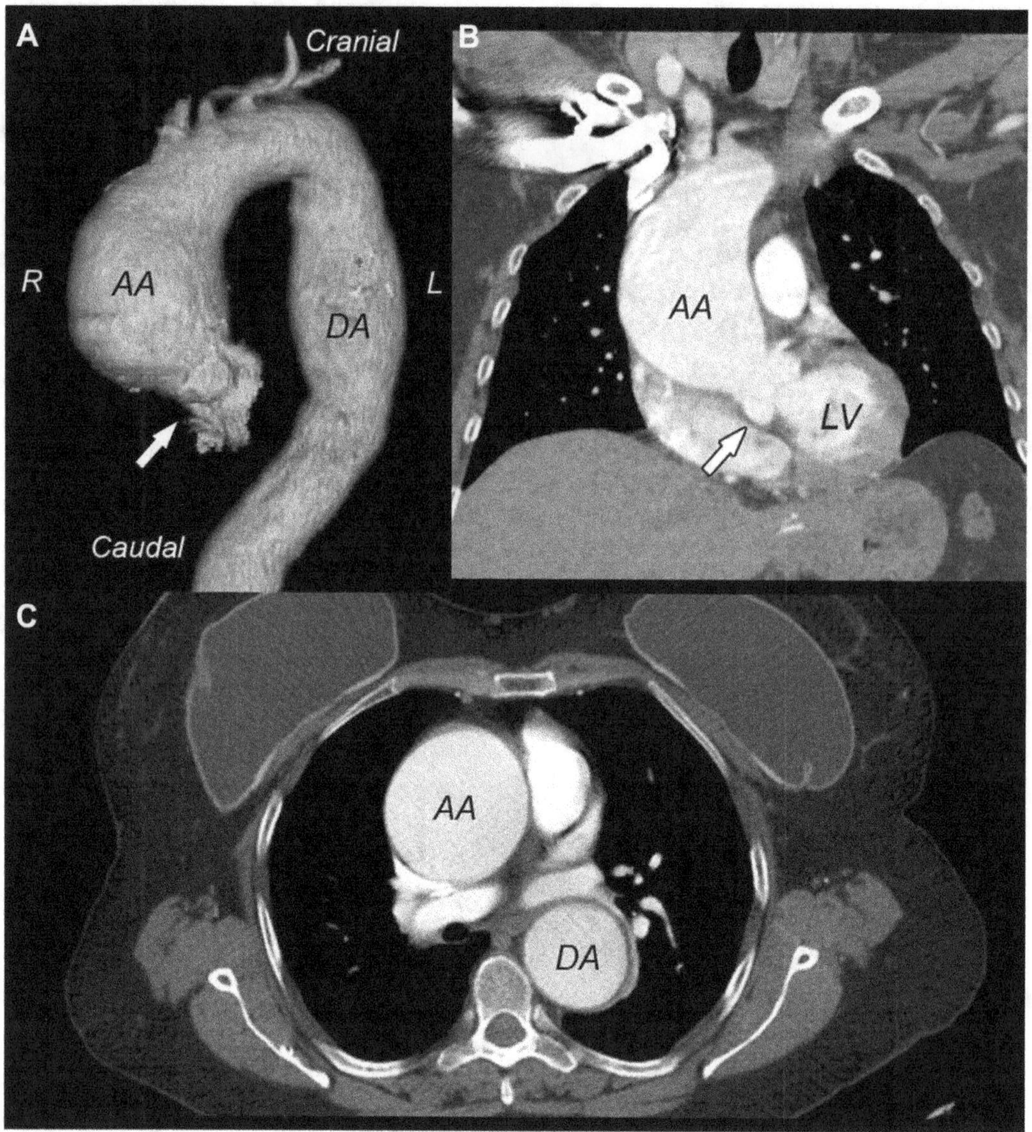



Figure 1. Patient #2, woman (Table 1). *(A)* Volume-rendered 3-dimensional reconstruction and *(B)* contrast-enhanced coronal and *(C)* axial CT images show a fusiform aneurysm of the AA and DA. The aortic sinuses are unaffected *(white arrows)*. The distal descending thoracic aorta is normal in caliber. AA = ascending aorta; DA = descending aorta; LV = left ventricular.

aneurysm. The aortic specimen in the 11 men ranged in weight from 14 to 46 g (mean 29) and in 11 of the 12 women from 11 to 27 g (mean 20). The 1 case not included in the weight of the aorta was a woman who had only a biopsy rather than resection of the aorta. Six patients also had aortic valve replacement because of pure aortic regurgitation. Their excised 3-cuspid valves weighed from 0.47 to 0.91 (mean 0.73, the normal aortic valve weighs ~0.50[6]). Coronary bypass also was performed at the time of ascending aortic resection in 6 patients (26%), and all 6 were ≥70 years of age.

An STS preoperatively was performed in 5 patients, and in only 1, the test result was positive. Some representative preoperative computed tomographic images and photographs of operatively excised ascending aortas are illustrated in Figures 1 to 4.

Histologic sections of the wall of the ascending aorta were similar in all 23 patients. All sections were stained by hematoxylin/eosin and by Movat methods, the latter to delineate the internal and external elastic membranes and the medial elastic fibers so that the intima, media, and adventitia could be clearly separated from one another.

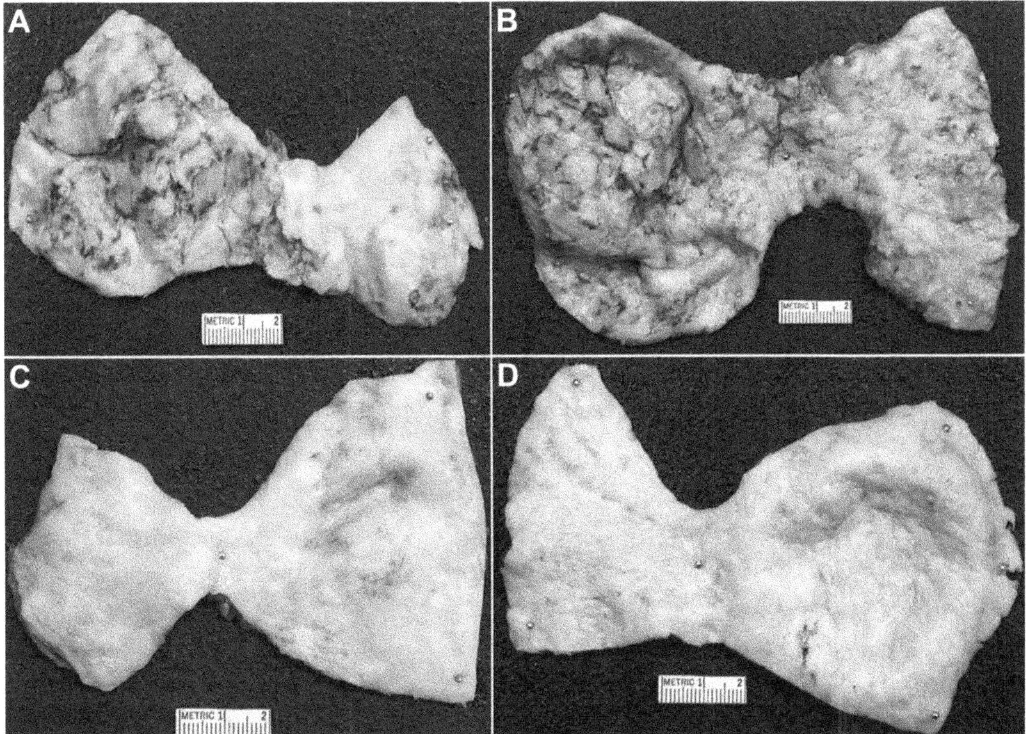

Figure 2. Excised ascending aortas in 4 patients, and arch is diffusely involved with the syphilitic process. *(A)* Case #1, man; *(B)* case #4, man; *(C)* case #8, man; *(D)* case #10, woman. *(A)* and *(B)* have extensive intimal calcific deposits, whereas *(C)* and *(D)* have no calcific deposits.

The wall of the aorta was thickened in all 23 patients because of thickening of the intima, mainly by fibrous tissue with or without calcific deposits, and by thickening of the adventitia by fibrous tissue within which were clumps of mononuclear cells (lymphocytes and plasmacytes). The vasa vasora in the adventitia were thickened, and the lumens of many were narrowed. The media was not thickened, but its elastic fibers were focally but extensively replaced by fibrous tissue. Occasionally, a few mononuclear cells were present in the media. Giant cells were absent.

## Comments

The major purpose of this report is to emphasize that syphilis remains a major cause of aneurysm of the ascending aorta with or without similar involvement of the arch and descending thoracic aorta. The 23 cases described here were seen in just over a 6-year period such that nearly 4 cases of syphilitic aortic aneurysms were resected at BUMC yearly.

Several decades ago, an STS was a requirement for admission to any US hospital. Today, an STS is infrequently performed in hospitalized patients in the United States. In 2004, the US Preventative Services Task Force found that there was no benefit in morbidity or mortality of screening for syphilis in asymptomatic adults or patients with high risk.[7] There are no studies, however, that evaluate the risks associated with screening and treating asymptomatic adult patients with syphilis. Given the morbidity associated with cardiovascular and neurologic syphilis, it is reasonable to do an STS in any patient with a 3-cuspid aortic valve and aneurysmal dilation of the ascending aorta with or without associated aortic regurgitation. Although there is a lack of randomized controlled trials, there is general consensus among the infectious disease community to treat patients with tertiary syphilis in an effort to prevent progression of the disease process. Unfortunately, the serologic test result for syphilis is often negative or nonreactive in patients with syphilitic aortitis, and thus, a negative result does not exclude this entity.[8]

Superimposition of a saccular aneurysm on a fusiform aneurysm of ascending aorta is virtually diagnostic of syphilitic aortitis. The syphilitic process begins at the sinotubular junction and spares the sinus portion of aorta, which, for example, is always involved in patients with the Marfan's syndrome or forme fruste varieties of that syndrome.[9,10]

Syphilis only involves the heart in a secondary manner. Aortic regurgitation in this entity is the consequence of the aortic dilation and not because of direct involvement of the

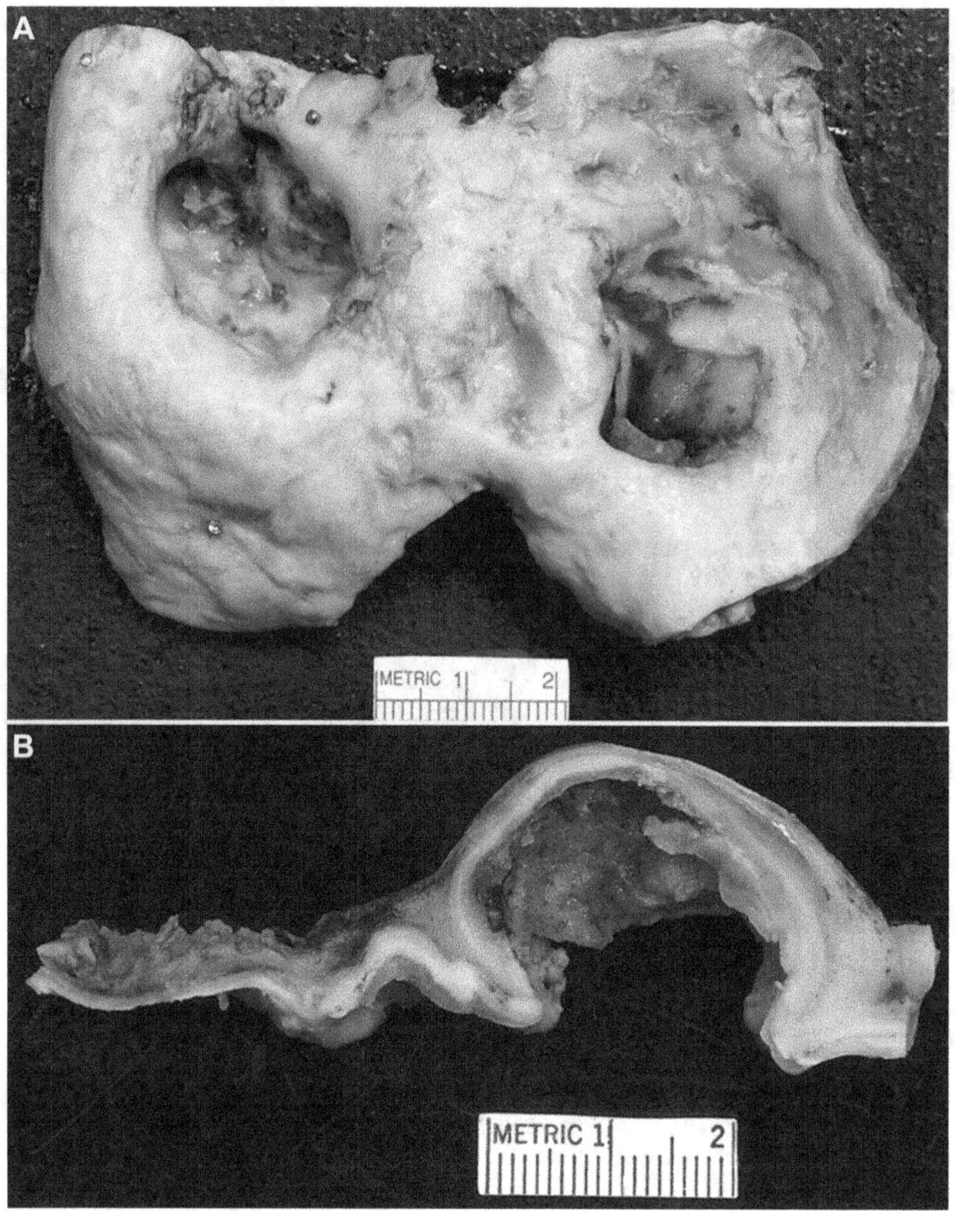

Figure 3. Case #3, man. *(A)* This resected ascending aorta contains 2 large saccular aneurysms arising from the fusiform aneurysm. *(B)* Cross-section of one of the saccular aneurysm partially filled with thrombus.

aortic valve cusps, the situation, for example, in ankylosing spondylitis that histologically is similar to syphilis, but this arthritic condition extends below (caudal to) the aortic valve, something syphilis never does. Additionally, syphilis never involves an epicardial coronary artery directly. Syphilis affects only the coronary ostia, nearly always the right one, and the narrowing is the result of the syphilitic process affecting the aorta, not the coronary artery directly. Consequently, it seems better to use the phrase "syphilitic aortitis" or "vascular syphilis" rather than the phrase "cardiovascular syphilis."

Syphilis is limited to the thoracic aorta and never involves the abdominal aorta.[11,12] The reason apparently is that vasa vasora are present only in the thoracic aorta, and they are absent in the abdominal aorta, and syphilis basically appears to be a disease of the vasa vasora, at least initially. Thus, when a fusiform abdominal aneurysm accompanies an ascending aortic aneurysm—in the

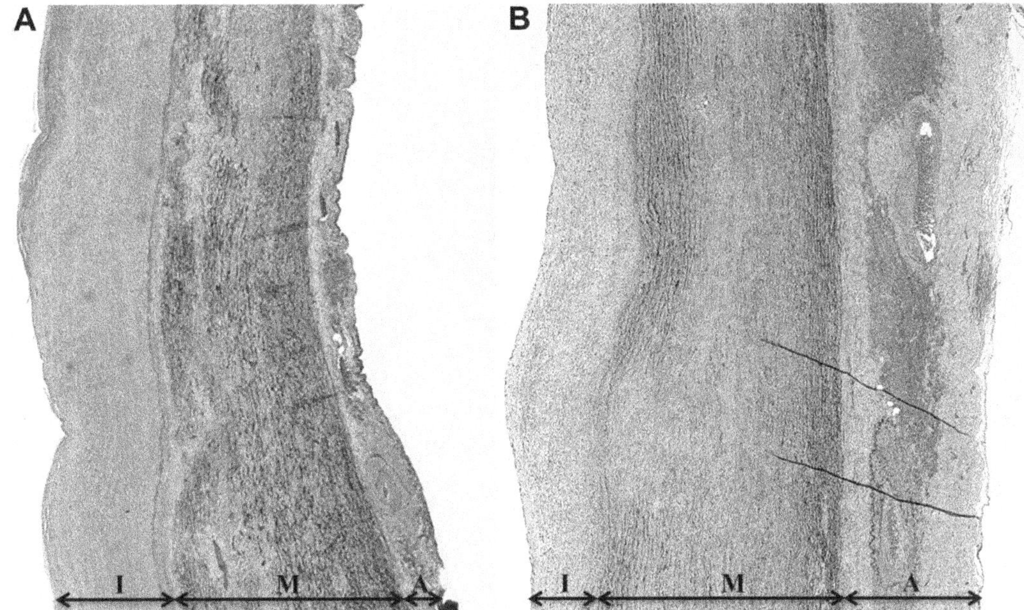


Figure 4. Photomicrographs of portions of ascending aorta in 2 patients. *(A)* Case #8, woman (Table 1). *(B)* Case #11, woman (Table 1). In each, the intima (I) and adventitia (A) are thickened, mainly by fibrous tissue. The adventitia contains large collections of lymphocytes and plasmacytes, shown best in *(B)*. The cells stain purple. The media (M) is not thickened, but many elastic fibers have been lost and replaced by fibrous tissue. Movat stains, ×40 *(A)*; ×40 *(B)*.

absence of aortic dissection—2 different processes are at work.

## Disclosures

The authors have no conflicts of interest to disclose.

1. Roberts WC, Bose R, Ko JM, Henry AC, Hamman BL. Identifying cardiovascular syphilis at operation. *Am J Cardiol* 2009;104: 1588–1594.
2. Roberts WC, Wibin EA. Idiopathic panaortitis, supraaortic arteritis, granulomatous myocarditis and pericarditis. A cause of pulseless disease and possibly left ventricular aneurysm in the African. *Am J Med* 1966;41:453–461.
3. Roberts WC, Zafar S, Ko JM. Morphological features of temporal arteritis. *Proc (Bayl Univ Med Cent)* 2013;26:109–115.
4. Bulkley BH, Roberts WC. Ankylosing spondylitis and aortic regurgitation: description of the characteristic cardiovascular lesion from study of eight necropsy patients. *Circulation* 1973;48:1014–1027.
5. Roberts WC, Hollingsworth JF, Bulkley BH, Jaffe RB, Epstein SE, Stinson EB. Combined mitral and aortic regurgitation in ankylosing spondylitis: angiographic and anatomic features. *Am J Med* 1974;56: 237–243.
6. Silver MA, Roberts WC. Detailed anatomy of the normally functioning aortic valve in hearts of normal and increased weight. *Am J Cardiol* 1985;55:454–461.
7. Calonge N; U.S. Preventive Services Task Force. Screening for syphilis infection: recommendation statement. *Ann Fam Med* 2004;2: 362–365.
8. Hart G. Syphilis tests in diagnostic and therapeutic decision making. *Ann Intern Med* 1986;104:368–376.
9. Waller BF, Reis RL, McIntosh CL, Epstein SE, Roberts WC. Marfan cardiovascular disease without the Marfan syndrome. *Chest* 1980;77: 533–540.
10. Roberts WC, Honig HS. The spectrum of cardiovascular disease in the Marfan syndrome: a clinico-morphologic study of 18 necropsy patients and comparison to 151 previously reported necropsy patients. *Am Heart J* 1982;104:115–135.
11. Roberts WC, Lensing FD, Kourlis H Jr, Ko JM, Newberry JW, Smerud MJ, Burton EC, Hebeler RF Jr. Full blown cardiovascular syphilis with aneurysm of the innominate artery. *Am J Cardiol* 2009;104: 1595–1600.
12. Wolinsky H, Glagov S. Nature of species differences in the medial distribution of aortic vasa vasorum in mammals. *Circ Res* 1967;20:409–421.

# Computed Tomographic and Morphologic Features of Syphilis of the Aorta

Clay M. Barbin, MD[a], Matthew R. Weissenborn, MD[b], Jong M. Ko, BA[c], Joseph E. Guileyardo, MD[d], and William C. Roberts, MD[a,c,d,*]

This report describes certain computed tomographic and morphologic features of syphilitic aortitis in 2 patients in whom the process involved the entire thoracic aorta. © 2015 Elsevier Inc. All rights reserved. (Am J Cardiol 2015;116:1311−1314)

In 2009, a report from this institution described certain necropsy features in 90 unoperated patients seen in a 25-year period with syphilis involving the aorta.[1] That report was the first to analyze characteristic features of vascular syphilis since 1964.[2] During a recent 4-month period, we studied at necropsy 2 additional patients with this condition, and the findings in them were unusual enough, in our view, to prompt this report.

## Description of Patients

Certain findings in each of the 2 patients are summarized in Table 1 and illustrated in Figures 1 to 3. Patient #1 had her aneurysmal ascending aorta resected and the aortic valve replaced (bi-leaflet mechanical valve-Carbomedics) at age 68. During the next 10 years, the descending thoracic aorta progressively enlarged. Seventeen days before death, a 36-cm-long stent was placed in the descending thoracic aorta. Postoperatively, movement in the legs progressively decreased and cardiac arrest occurred. The mechanical valve in the aortic-valve position appeared to have functioned properly (This patient was on warfarin chronically.). At necropsy, nearly 2,000 ml of blood was found in the right pleural space, and a rupture site was seen at the bend in the thoracic aorta.

Patient #2 collapsed at home, and the paramedics found him to have pulseless electrical activity. He was brought to the emergency room, had another cardiac arrest, and died. Necropsy disclosed a large ruptured fusiform abdominal aortic aneurysm.

Both patients had fusiform aneurysms involving the entire thoracic aorta with multiple saccular aneurysms, most containing thrombus, arising from the diffusely dilated aorta. Histologic study of the walls of the thoracic aortic aneurysms disclosed typical findings of syphilis: fibrous thickening of the adventitia containing foci of lymphocytes and plasmacytes and thickened vasa vasora, thickened intima by fibrous plaque with focal calcific deposits, and

Table 1
Certain clinical and necropsy findings in the 2 patients with syphilis of the aorta

| Variable | Patient | |
| --- | --- | --- |
| | #1 | #2 |
| Age (years) | 78 | 71 |
| Gender | Female | Male |
| Race | Black | White |
| Highest blood pressure (mm Hg) | 180/90 | 145/80 |
| Hypertension (history) | + | + |
| Aortic regurgitation | + | o |
| Obesity | + | + |
| Heart weight (g) | 565 | 410 |
| Operation, aorta | + | o |
| Stent, aorta | + | o |
| Cause of death | Rupture, DTA | Rupture, AAA |
| Cardiac adiposity* | + | + |

AAA = abdominal aortic aneurysm; DTA = descending thoracic aorta.
* Both hearts floated in a container of formaldehyde.

nonthickened media with focal but massive loss of elastic fibers. Neither patient had significant narrowing of the epicardial coronary arteries themselves, neither had grossly visible myocardial lesions, and neither had dilated cardiac ventricles.

Serologic and molecular tests for syphilis (antibody treponema palladium and polymerase chain reactive) on postmortem blood were nonreactive or not detectable in both patients.

## Comments

Each of the hitherto described patients had large fusiform aneurysms involving the entire thoracic aorta with multiple saccular aneurysms originating from the wall of the fusiform aneurysm. Each died from rupture of the aorta: one (case #1) of the descending thoracic aorta into which had been inserted a long (36 cm) metallic stent and one (case #2) of a fusiform abdominal aorta aneurysm, something unrelated to the syphilitic aneurysm of the thoracic aorta. Although histologic study of the thoracic aorta in each patient was classic of syphilis (fibrous thickening of the adventitia containing focal collections of plasmacytes and lymphocytes and thickened vasa vasora, fibrous thickening of the intima containing focal calcific deposits, and massive loss of medial elastic fibers with replacement by fibrous tissue), serologic and molecular test results for syphilis on postmortem blood were negative or nonreactive in both patients. (The serologic test results for syphilis are often negative in

Departments of [a]Internal Medicine, [b]Radiology, [d]Pathology, and [c]Baylor Heart and Vascular Institute, Baylor University Medical Center, Dallas, Texas. Manuscript received June 30, 2015; revised manuscript received and accepted July 3, 2015.

The study was funded by the Baylor Health Care System Foundation, Dallas,Texas.

See page 1314 for disclosure information.

*Corresponding author: Tel: (214) 820-7911; fax: (214) 820-7533.

*E-mail address:* wc.roberts@baylorhealth.edu (W.C. Roberts).

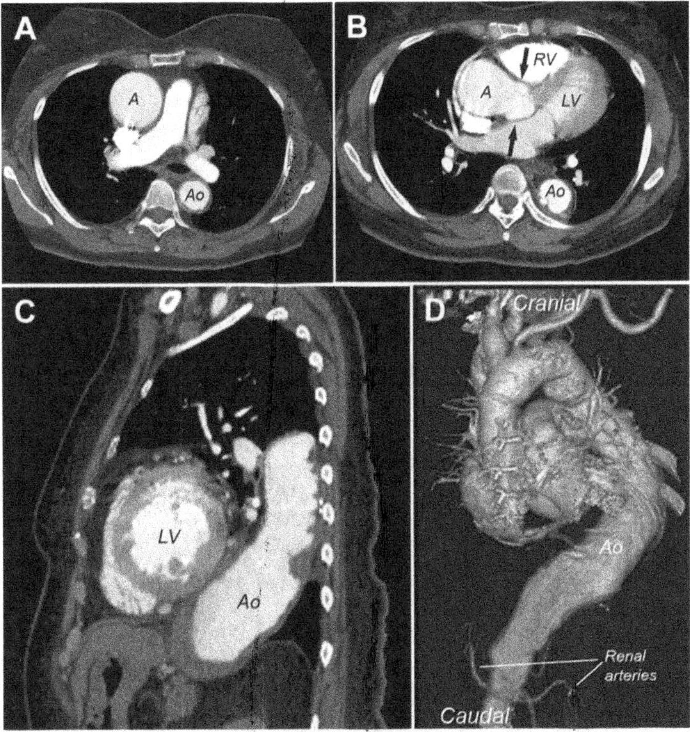

Figure 1. Case #1. *(A and B)* Contrast-enhanced computed tomographic axial images before aortic valve replacement for aortic regurgitation 10 years before death showing a fusiform aneurysm of the ascending aorta with mural calcific deposits. The aortic sinus *(black arrows)* is not dilated. *(C)* Contrast-enhanced sagittal computed tomographic image shortly before death revealing a fusiform aneurysm of the descending aorta with atherosclerotic plaque formation. *(D)* Volume-rendered 3-dimensional reconstruction showing the fusiform aneurysm of the descending aorta replacement. The patient 10 years earlier had resection of the ascending aortic aneurysm, replacement of the aortic valve, and resection of the ascending aorta. A = ascending aorta, Ao = descending aorta, LV = left ventricular cavity, RV = right ventricular cavity.

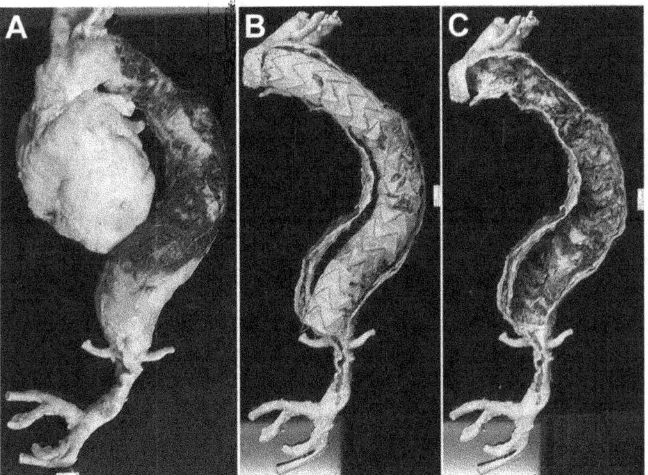

Figure 2. Case #1. Views of the heart and aorta at necropsy. *(A)* The heart and the entire aorta. The ascending portion contains a graft. Both the arch and descending portions are diffusely dilated. Blood is present in the adventitia because of its rupture in the area of the bend. The diameter of the abdominal aorta is normal (∼ 1.5 cm). *(B)* The aorta is "de-roofed" exposing the 36-cm stent. *(C)* The stent has been removed exposing the interior lining. The wall of the aorta in most portions is thickened.

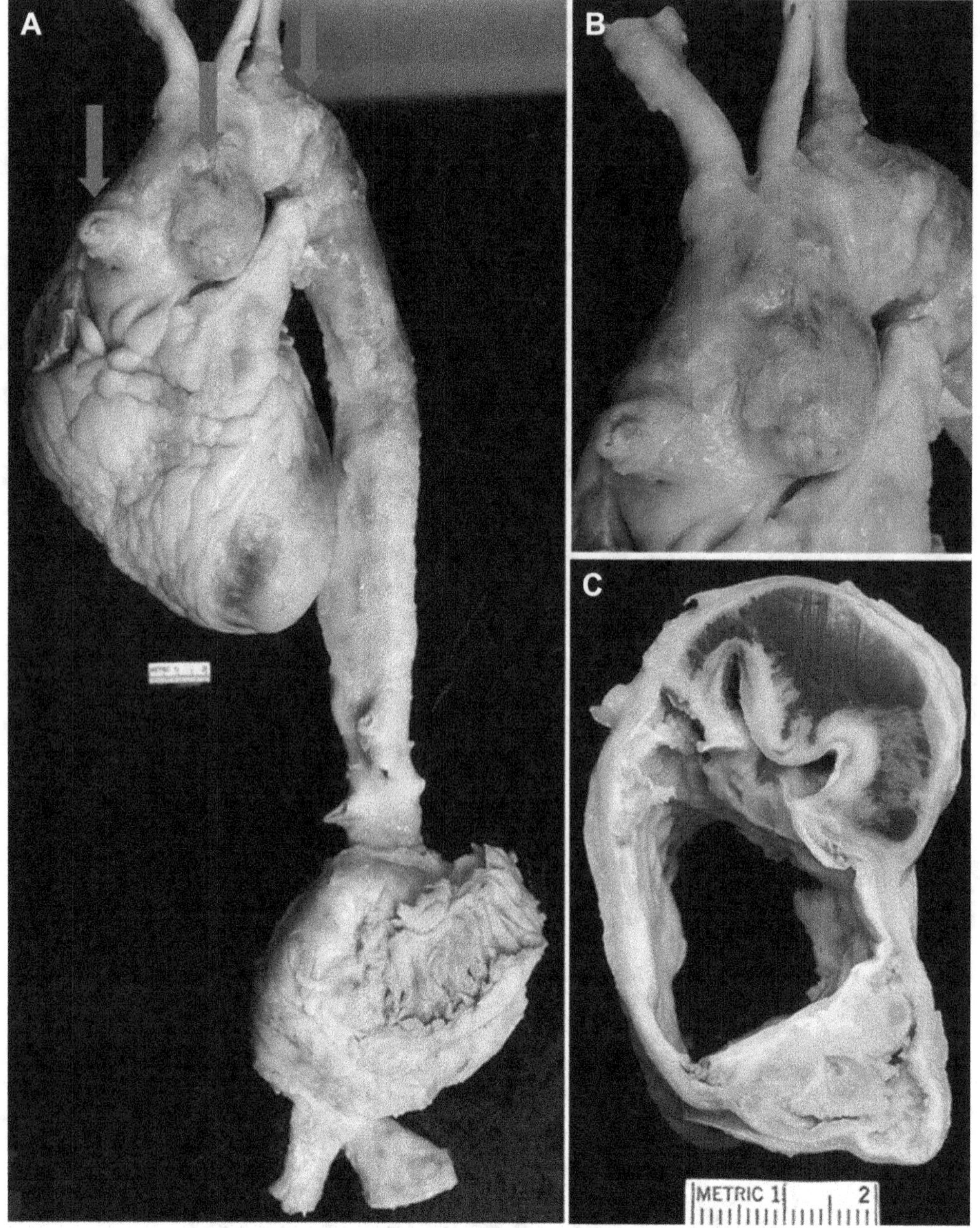

Figure 3. Case #2. Heart and aorta. *(A)* Several saccular[3] aneurysms *(arrows)* protrude from the fusiform aneurysm involving all portions of the thoracic aorta. The fusiform aneurysm in the abdominal portion is attached to the duodenum. The aorta just cephalad to the abdominal aneurysm is of normal diameter. *(B)* Close-up view of the multiple saccular aneurysms involving the ascending and arch portions of aorta. *(C)* Two saccular aneurysms arising from the ascending aorta. Thrombus fills one of them and lipid plaque fills the other.

patients with typical syphilitic involvement of the aorta.[1,2,4,5])

Although computed tomographic imaging of aneurysmally dilated aortas is a common occurrence, such procedures in patients with histologically confirmed syphilitic aortitis have been infrequent. Another unusual feature was the insertion of the stent in the entire descending thoracic aorta in patient #1. In retrospect that procedure was risky because the patient was on long-term warfarin therapy for the mechanical prosthesis in the aortic valve position (inserted 10 years earlier). Although patient #1 had had aortic regurgitation, this dysfunction was a complication of the involvement of the aorta by the syphilitic process and not a primary cardiac abnormality. Indeed, neither patient had significant atherosclerosis of the epicardial coronary arteries or grossly visible myocardial lesions or dilation of either ventricular cavity. Thus, actual involvement of the heart in syphilis in our view is a nonentity. Syphilis of the vascular system means involvement only of the thoracic aorta and its branches. The phrase "cardiovascular syphilis" might better be replaced by the phrase "syphilis of the aorta" or "aortic syphilis."

Although patient #2 had a large abdominal aortic aneurysm, its etiology was not syphilis, which has never been reported to involve the abdominal aorta. The reason appears to be the lack of vasa vasora in the abdominal aorta, which normally possesses about 28 elastic lamellae in the media.[6] The ascending aorta, in contrast, contains about 56 elastic lamellae in its media and the vasa vasora penetrate its outer half or the outer 28 elastic lamellae.[6] Because the abdominal aorta contains only 28 elastic lamellae, its wall is perfused entirely by blood in the aorta's lumen and vasa vasora are unnecessary.

## Disclosures

The authors have no conflicts of interest to disclose.


1. Roberts WC, Ko JM, Vowels TJ. Natural history of syphilitic aortitis. *Am J Cardiol* 2009;104:1578–1587.
2. Heggtveit HA. Syphilitic aortitis. A clinicopathologic autopsy study of 100 cases, 1950 to 1960. *Circulation* 1964;29:346–355.
3. Beckh W. The serologic reaction in cardiovascular syphilis. *Am Heart J* 1943;24:307–312.
4. Atwoo WG, Miller JL, Stout GW, Norins LC. The TPI and FTA-ABS tests in treated late syphilis. *JAMA* 1968;203:549–551.
5. Gormsen H. Postmortem diagnosis of syphilitic aortitis, including serological verification on postmortem blood. *Forensic Sci Int* 1984;24:51–56.
6. Wolinky H, Glagov S. Nature of species differences in the medial distribution of aortic vasa vasorum in mammals. *Circ Res* 1967;20:409–421.

# Operative Recognition of Syphilis of the Aorta

William C. Roberts, MD*, and Nitin Kondapalli, MBBS

**Aortic syphilis has not disappeared. Few patients with aortic syphilis are diagnosed preoperatively or after histologic examination of the resected aortas. The gross features of the wall of the syphilitic aortic aneurysm, however, are unique allowing diagnosis of this entity on the operating table. Thirty patients aged 33 to 84 years (mean 66) (18 women) had a syphilitic aneurysm involving the tubular portion of ascending aorta resected at Baylor University Medical Center at Dallas from 2009 through 2017. That syphilis was the cause of the aneurysm was not appreciated either preoperatively or at operation. Syphilis produces characteristic changes in the aorta: it is thicker than normal due to fibrous thickening of the intima and adventitia, the intimal surface is 100% abnormal, and the sinus portion of the aorta is uninvolved. The process begins at or just distal to the sinotubular junction. Histologic findings are specific. A negative serologic test for syphilis does not rule out the presence of syphilis of the aorta. The key to identifying at operation syphilis of the aorta is to note that its entire intimal surface is abnormal, that one or more saccular aneurysms may arise from the fusiform aneurysm, that the aneurysmal wall is thicker than normal, and that the wall of the sinus portion of the aorta is spared. Identification of the syphilitic cause appears to be important because antibiotic therapy is recommended to prevent or retard the development of neurological syphilis, particularly in the younger patients.** © 2018 Elsevier Inc. All rights reserved. (Am J Cardiol 2018;122:898−904)

In the last 10 years we have published several articles on syphilis of the aorta including an article entitled "Identifying Cardiovascular Syphilis at Operation".[1-6] The latter article described 34 patients seen in the previous 50 years (1958 - 2008) with aneurysmal ascending aortas and histological study of the walls of the resected aneurysms disclosed classic syphilis.[1] None of the 34 patients had had cardiovascular syphilis diagnosed preoperatively. Subsequently, one of us (WCR) interviewed a prominent cardiovascular surgeon particularly interested in the thoracic aorta and he indicated that despite excising numerous aneurysms of the ascending aorta in St. Louis, Rochester and Boston that he had never encountered cardiovascular syphilis.[7] Since our report in 2009, we have subsequently studied 30 additional patients in whom classic syphilitic aneurysms were resected, and the syphilitic cause of the aneurysm was not recognized at operation in any patient. Because of the poor recognition of aortic syphilis at operation, we prepared this additional report in hopes of bringing some focus to this returning disease of the aorta.

Baylor Heart and Vascular Institute, the Departments of Pathology and Internal Medicine (Division of Cardiology), Baylor University Medical Center, Dallas, Texas. Manuscript received May 1, 2018; revised manuscript received and accepted May 4, 2018.

See page 903 for disclosure information.

*Corresponding Author: William C. Roberts, MD. Baylor Heart and Vascular Institute, Baylor University Medical Center, 621 N. Hall Street, Suite H-030, Dallas, Texas 75226. Tel.: 011 214 820 7911.

*E-mail addresses:* William.Roberts1@bswhealth.org, ajc@baylorhealth.edu (W.C. Roberts).

## Methods

Pertinent data in each of the 30 patients is presented in Table 1: their ages ranged from 33 to 84 years (mean 66); 18 were women (60%), and 12 were men (40%). Aortic regurgitation (ranging from 1+ to 4+) was present in 19 patients (63%), 7 of whom had concomitant aortic valve replacement. The largest diameter of the ascending aortic aneurysm (known in 29 patients) preoperatively ranged from 4.3 to 8.2 cm (mean 5.6), and in 26 (90%) it was >4.5 cm. A serological test for syphilis was done in 8 patients: preoperatively in 4, and it was positive in 1; postoperatively, in 4 others and it was non-reactive in all 4. A serologic test for AIDS was performed in 3 patients and it was negative in all 3. None of the other 27 patients were known to have AIDS. Seven (23%) of the 30 patients had a body mass index >30 Kg/m$^2$.

The resected aortas and aortic valves in all 30 patients was submitted to the surgical pathology section of the department of pathology of Baylor University Medical Center. All were examined and the report prepared by one of us (WCR). All specimens were photographed (by Saba Ilyas), weighed (by WCR), and histological sections prepared. Both an elastic tissue stain (Movat) and a hematoxylin/eosin stain were prepared on all sections of aorta, and all sections were examined by WCR, usually about 20 cm of Movat stained sections in each patient. The exception was patient #14 where only a biopsy of the wall of the aneurysm was performed.

The clinical records in all 30 patients were reviewed and certain findings in them are tabulated in Table 1.

Table 1
Clinical and morphological findings in 30 patients who underwent resection of ascending aorta for cardiovascular syphilis (ascending aortic aneurysm with or without aortic regurgitation) arranged according to age at aortic operation

| Pt. No. | Age (years) at Operation | Sex | Race | Peak Systolic/ End Diastolic Pressure (mm Hg) | | AR (0-4+) | STS done (type) | STS result | BMI (kg/m2) | Year of Operation | AA Weight (g) | AVR (AV Weight) | CABG | Diameter in cm of Fusiform Ascending Aortic Aneurysm (type image) | Saccular Aneurysm | Interval Between Operation and Death |
|---|---|---|---|---|---|---|---|---|---|---|---|---|---|---|---|---|
| | | | | LV | AA | | | | | | | | | | | |
| 1 | 33 | M | W | 118/27 | 132/73 | 3+ | 0 | - | 25 | 2010 | 16 | +(0.47g) | 0 | 5.7(CT) | 0 | - |
| 2 | 36 | F | W | 131/8 | 129/70 | 2+ | +(TPPA) | NR | 20 | 2017 | 21 | +(0.51g) | 0 | 4.9(CT) | 0 | - |
| 3 | 45 | M | B | - | 135/95[a] | 0 | +(TPPA)[e] | R[f] | 21 | 2013 | 32 | 0 | 0 | 8.2(CT) | + | - |
| 4 | 48 | M | B | - | 106/65[a] | 0 | 0 | - | 28 | 2012 | 46 | 0 | 0 | 6.2(CT) | + | - |
| 5 | 51 | M | W | 148/20 | 131/60 | 1+ | 0 | - | 29 | 2009 | 42 | 0 | 0 | 7.4(MRA) | 0 | - |
| 6 | 52 | F | W | - | 105/65[a] | 0 | 0 | - | 25 | 2015 | 23 | 0 | 0 | 5.9(CT) | 0 | - |
| 7 | 58 | F | B | 126/3 | 140/90[a] | 0 | 0 | - | 32 | 2013 | 11 | 0 | 0 | 5.1(Echo) | 0 | - |
| 8 | 59 | F | W | - | 156/83 | 0 | 0 | - | 30 | 2010 | 27 | 0 | 0 | 6.6(CT) | 0 | - |
| 9 | 59 | M | A | - | 170/80[a] | 2+ | 0 | - | 28 | 2014 | 44 | 0 | 0 | 4.6(CT) | + | 1 day |
| 10 | 60 | M | W | 120/7 | 121/65 | 0 | 0 | - | 29 | 2013 | 22 | 0 | 0 | 5.6(CT) | 0 | - |
| 11 | 62 | F | W | 155/25 | 170/65 | 4+ | +(RPR) | NR | 46 | 2012 | 14 | +(0.78g) | 0 | 5.1(CT) | + | - |
| 12 | 65 | F | W | 114/16 | 117/67 | 0 | 0 | - | 36 | 2009 | 22 | 0 | 0 | 4.5(Echo) | 0 | - |
| 13 | 65 | F | W | 153/13 | 154/83 | 0 | 0 | - | 29 | 2009 | 22 | 0 | 0 | 4.3(CT) | 0 | - |
| 14 | 67 | F | W | 124/4 | 135/60 | 3+ | +(RPR)[e] | NR | 26 | 2013 | 0.1[b] | 0[d] | 0 | "Dilated" | 0 | - |
| 15 | 69 | F | W | 101/1 | 101/51 | 0 | 0 | - | 15 | 2012 | 24 | 0 | + | 5.6(CT) | 0 | - |
| 16 | 69 | M | W | 164/-2 | 168/62 | 2+ | +(TPPA)[e] | NR | 34 | 2016 | 27 | +(0.69g) | 0 | 6.6(CT) | 0 | - |
| 17 | 69 | F | W | - | 105/65[a] | 0 | 0 | - | 32 | 2016 | 17 | 0 | + | 5.0(CT) | 0 | - |
| 18 | 70 | M | W | 173/33 | 170/71 | 2+ | 0 | - | 38 | 2011 | 22 | 0 | + | 4.5(Echo) | 0 | - |
| 19 | 70 | F | W | - | 135/60[a] | 0 | +(RPR) | NR | 19 | 2011 | 25 | 0 | 0 | 5.4(CT) | 0 | - |
| 20 | 72 | F | W | - | 120/65[a] | 2+ | 0 | - | 38 | 2016 | 26 | 0 | 0[e] | 5.7(CT) | 0 | 13 months |
| 21 | 72 | F | W | - | 115/55[a] | 2+ | 0 | - | 31 | 2017 | 19 | 0 | 0 | 6.0(CT) | 0 | - |
| 22 | 74 | M | B | - | 175/85[a] | 1+ | 0 | - | 25 | 2017 | 33 | 0 | 0 | 6.1(CT) | 0 | - |
| 23 | 76 | F | W | 106/1 | 109/44 | 1+ | +(TPPA)[e] | NR | 30 | 2016 | 25 | 0 | 0 | 4.8(Echo) | 0 | - |
| 24 | 77 | F | W | 204/34 | 190/88 | 2+ | 0 | - | 28 | 2017 | 24 | 0[d] | 0 | 5.5(CT) | 0 | 2 months |
| 25 | 80 | F | W | 144/27 | 140/54 | 2+ | +(RPR) | NR | 29 | 2010 | 20 | 0 | 0 | 5.5(CT) | 0 | - |
| 26 | 80 | M | W | 129/9 | 130/59 | 2+ | 0 | - | 28 | 2012 | 22 | 0 | + | 6.1(CT) | 0 | - |
| 27 | 83 | M | W | 130/10 | 150/80 | 3+ | 0 | - | 24 | 2010 | 27 | +(0.91g) | + | 5.8(CT) | 0 | 92 months |
| 28 | 83 | F | W | 124/13 | 123/58 | 1+ | 0 | - | 23 | 2010 | 21 | 0 | 0 | 5.8(CT) | 0 | - |
| 29 | 83 | F | W | 182/86 | 179/54 | 3+ | 0 | - | 19 | 2011 | 13 | +(0.55g) | 0 | 5.0(Echo) | 0 | 71 months |
| 30 | 84 | M | W | 121/19 | 103/63 | 2+ | 0 | - | 27 | 2009 | 29 | +(0.86g) | + | 6.1(CT) | 0 | 43 months |
| Range (Mean) | 33-84 (66) | | | | | | | | 15-46(28) | | 11-46(25) | 0.47-0.91(0.64) | | 4.3-8.2(5.6) | | |

A. = Asian; AA = Ascending Aorta; AR = Aortic Regurgitation; AV = Aortic Valve; AVR = Aortic Valve Replacement; B = Black; BMI = Body Mass Index; cm = centimeters; CABG = Coronary Artery Bypass Grafting; CT = Computerized Tomography; Echo = Echocardiography; F = Female; g = gram(s); LV = Left Ventricle; MRA = Magnetic Resonance Angiography; M = Male; NR = Nonreactive; Pt. No. = Patient Number; PCI = Percutaneous Coronary Intervention; RPR = Rapid Plasma Reagin test; R = Reactive; STS = Serological Test for Syphilis; TPPA = Treponema Pallidum Particle Agglutination assay; W = White; - = no information available.

[a] Indirect pressure (cuff)

[b] Only a biopsy of aorta was performed. It weighed only 0.1g. This weight was not included in the average for the other 29 patients

[c] Percutaneous coronary intervention done

[d] Aortic valve repair done

[e] STS test done operation

[f] Reactive treponemal antibody test - confirmed by RPR at 1:128 dilution.

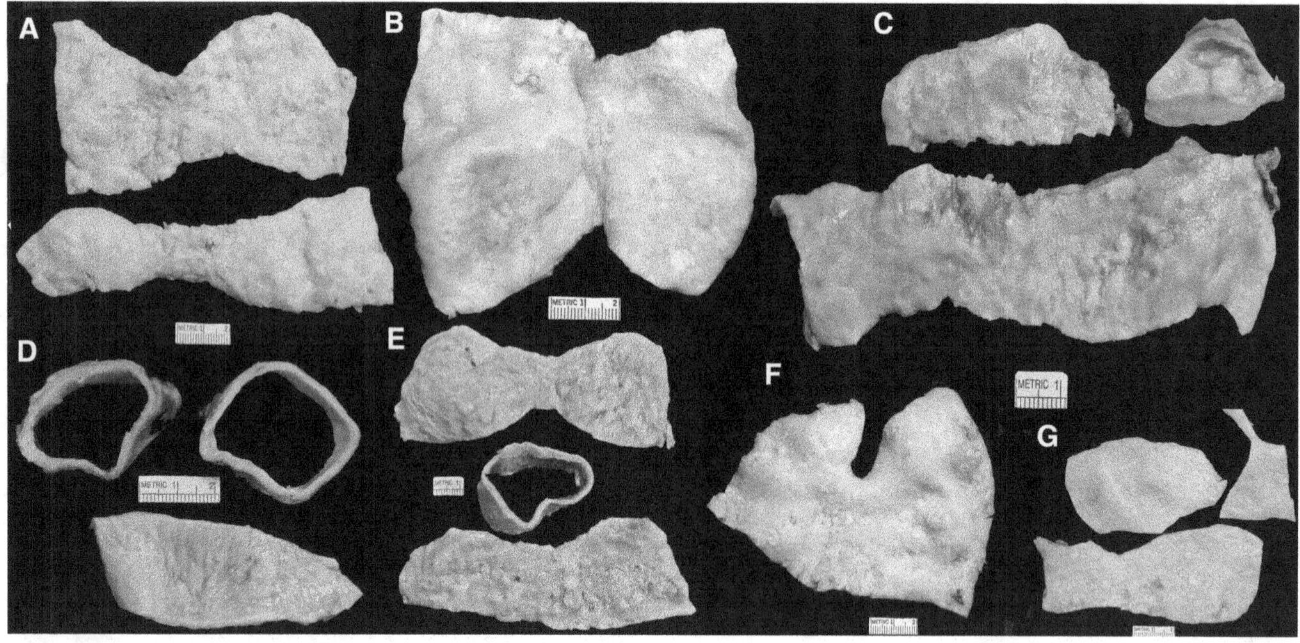

Fig. 1. Shown here are the excised portions of the tubular portion of ascending aorta in 7 patients. Every square millimeter of the surface in each of these 7 patients is abnormal. *(A):* patient #6; *(B):* patient #15; *(C):* ) patient #20; *(D):* patient #21; *(E):* patient #23; *(F):* patient #26, and *(G):* patient #28. In *(D)* and *(E)* an intact portion of aorta is also shown.

## Results

All 30 patients included herein had classic histological features of syphilis of the aorta: the wall of the aneurysm was much thicker than normal due to increased thickness of the intima and the adventitia, mainly by fibrous tissue; within the thickened adventitia were focal collections of mononuclear cells, namely lymphocytes and plasmacytes; the walls of the vasa vasora in the adventitia were thickened and their lumens were narrowed (by fibrous tissue); numerous elastic fibers in the media were absent and replaced by fibrous tissue, and occasionally a few monocytes were present in the media (Figures 1-8). All patients in this study fulfilled these histologic criteria for aortic syphilis. Saccular aneurysms arose from the wall of the fusiform aneurysm in the ascending aorta in 4 (13%) of the 30 cases.

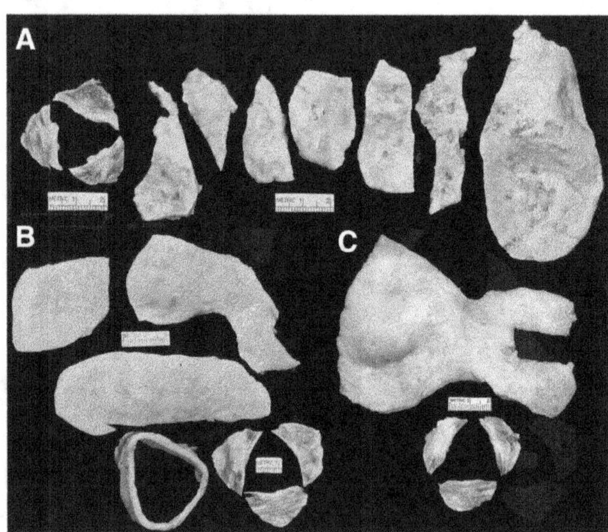

Fig. 2. Shown here are excised portions of ascending aorta and the excised aortic valves in 3 patients. Again, every square millimeter of the aorta is abnormal. The aortic valves are normal except for mild fibrous thickening of the free margin, mainly in the central portion. *(A):* patient #2; *(B):* patient #16; and *(C):* patient #27.

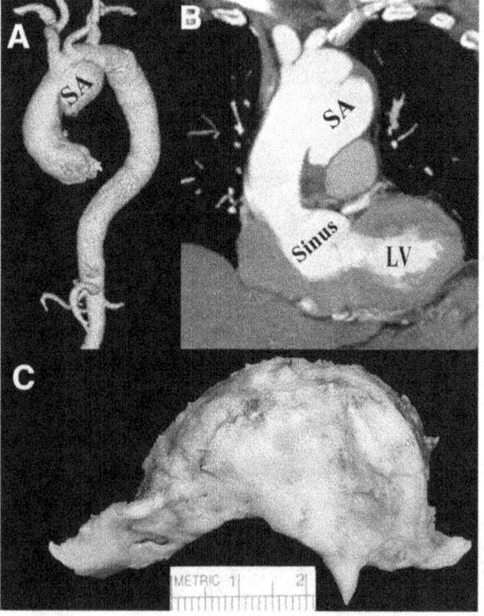

Fig. 3. Patient #9. *(A):* A computed tomographic image of most of the aorta showing a saccular aneurysm (SA) protruding on the caudal portion of aorta at the beginning of the arch. *(B):* A different view of the saccular aneurysm also showing the sinuses of Valsalva and the left ventricular (LV) cavity. *(C):* Wall of the saccular aneurysm (SA), the intimal surface of which is 100% abnormal.

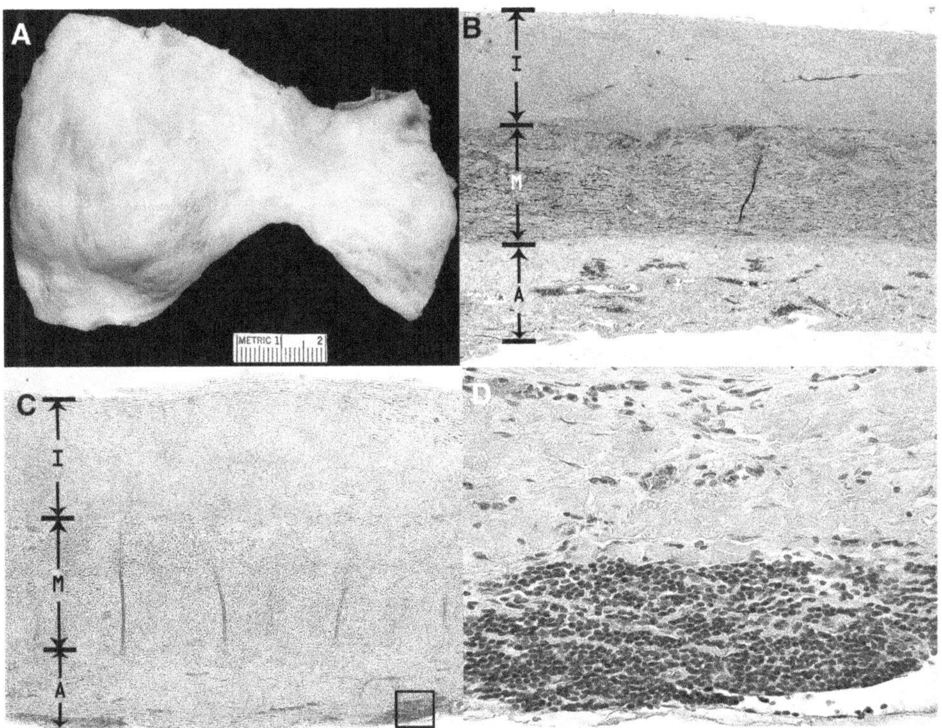

Fig. 4. Patient #10. *(A):* The resected portion of ascending aorta. Again, every square millimeter of the intimal surface is abnormal. *(B):* A Movat-stained section of a portion of aorta showing the intima (I) to be thickened by fibrous tissue; a focally-scarred media (M), and fibrous thickening of the adventitia (A). *(C):* A hematoxylin/eosin-stained section of aorta showing a collection of lymphocytes/plasmacytes in one portion of the outer adventitia. *(D):* A close-up view of the area shown in brackets in *(C)*. Movat stain, X40 *(B)*); hematoxylin/eosin stain, X40 *(C)* and X400 *(D)*.

## Comments

Identifying aortic syphilis by examining its aneurysmal wall by gross inspection is not difficult: every single millimeter of the intimal surface is abnormal! That situation is not produced in any other condition except homozygous familial hypercholesterolemia[8,9] and in that scenario the adventitia and media are usually normal. In syphilis the aortic wall is thicker than normal. The thickness is due to diffuse thickening of the intima, with or without focal calcific deposits, and to fibrous thickening of the adventitia which contains focal collections of plasmacytes and lymphocytes. The media is not thickened but its elastic fibers are interrupted by fibrous scars. The vasa vasora have thickened walls and narrowed lumens. Additionally, the only

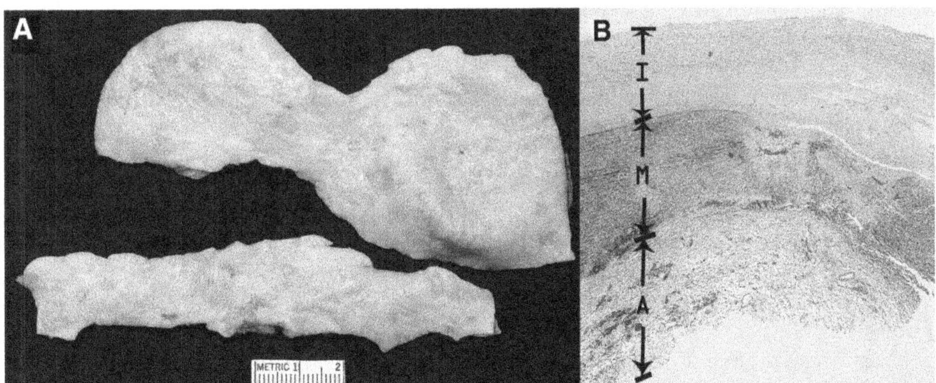

Fig. 5. Patient #12. *(A):* The excised portion of ascending aorta. Every square millimeter of the intimal surface is abnormal. *(B):* Photomicrograph of a section of aorta showing fibrous thickening of the intima (I), focal loss of elastic fibers in the media (M), and fibrous thickening of the adventitia (A) which contains foci of lymphocytes/plasmacytes. Movat stain, X 40 *(B)*.

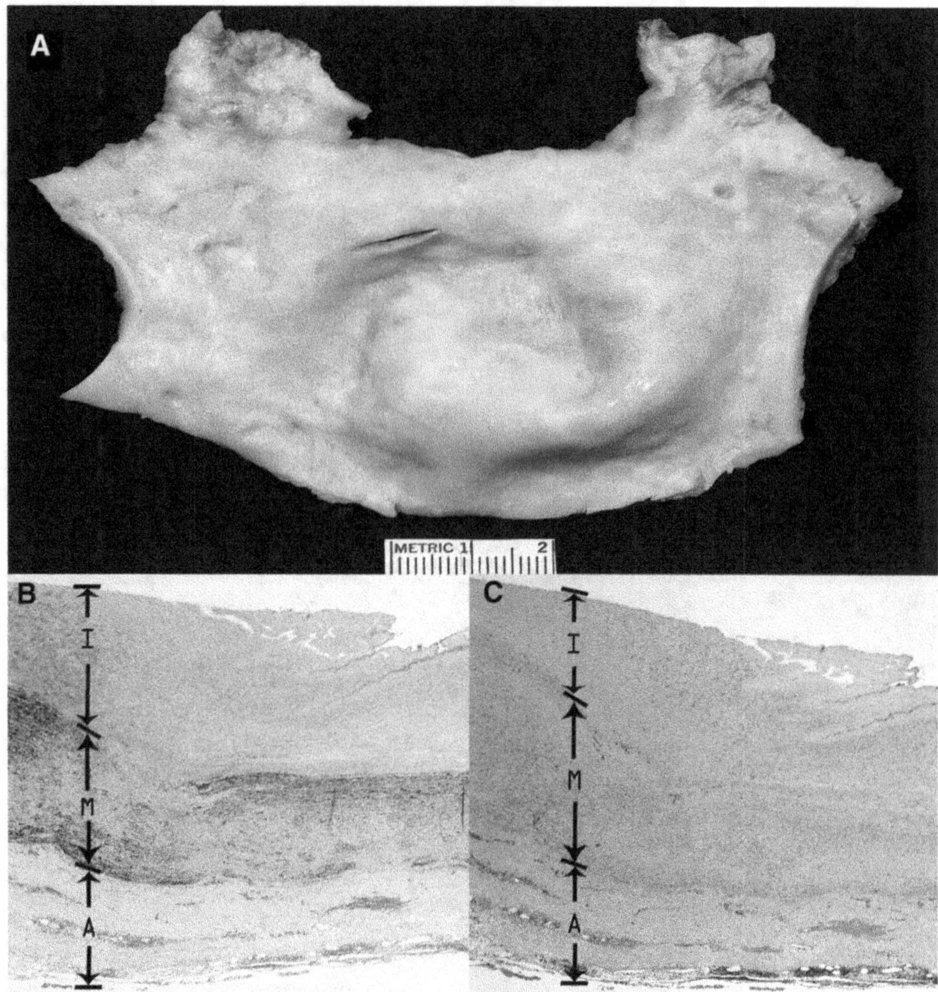

Fig. 6. Patient #13. *(A):* Resected portion of ascending aorta. Again, the entire intimal surface is abnormal. *(B):* A photomicrograph of a Movat-stained section showing marked thickening of the intima (I), marked scarring of the media (M), and fibrous thickening of the adventitia (A). *(C):* Roughly the same portion of aorta seen in *(B)* but stained by hematoxylin/eosin. The outer portion of the adventitia contains islands of lymphocytes/plasmacytes. Movat stain, X40 *(B)*; hematoxylin/eosin stain, X40 *(C)*.

portion of the ascending aorta involved by syphilis is the tubular portion; the sinus portion of the aorta is spared. The syphilitic process begins at the sinotubular junction or just cephalad to that junction. The entire wall of the tubular portion is involved by the syphilitic process. Additionally, one or more saccular aneurysms may arise from the wall of the fusiform aneurysm in the tubular portion of ascending aorta. On occasion, the syphilitic process may involve the arch and the descending thoracic aorta but never the abdominal aorta (because there are no vasa vasora in the abdominal aorta). Spirochetes have never been seen on histologic sections of ascending aorta in these patients. *Treponema pallidum* has never been cultured, to our knowledge, from resected aortas in patients with aortic syphilis (Figs. 1–8).

Recognition of aortic syphilis at the time of operation appears to be important for these patients who probably would benefit from a course of antibiotic therapy, primarily to prevent the occurrence of neurosyphilis and to prevent aortic progression. A serological test for syphilis is often negative in patients with demonstrated syphilis of the aorta as occurred in several patients included herein. If the process is not recognized either by the surgeon or by the surgical pathologist (now often unfamiliar with the histologic features of aortic syphilis) antibiotics will not be administered. Whether the antibiotic course would be useful to prevent or retard the extension of the syphilitic process to the arch or descending thoracic aorta or to prevent neurosyphilis, however, is unknown.

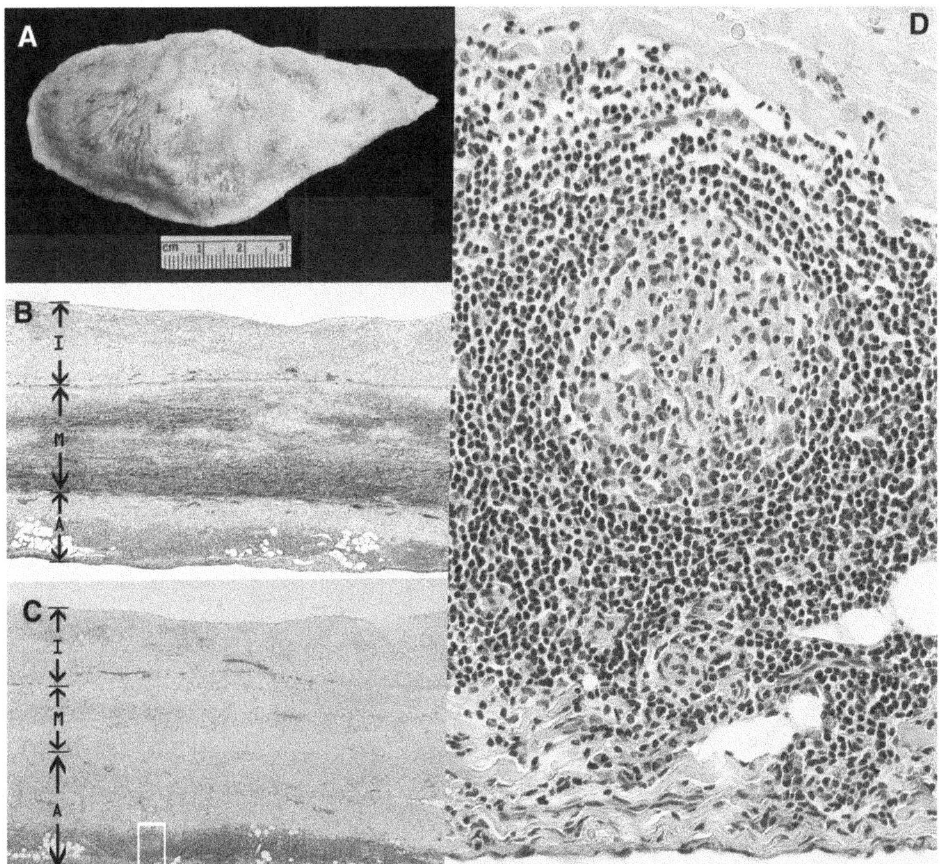

Fig. 7. Patient #17. *(A):* The resected portion of ascending aorta. Again, every square millimeter of the intima is abnormal. *(B):* A photomicrograph of a Movat-stained section of aorta showing a thickened intima (I), focal but extensive scarring of the media (M), and fibrous thickening of the adventitia (A). *(C):* A hematoxylin/eosin stained section of roughly the area shown in *(B)*. The adventitia contains huge collections of lymphocytes/plasmacytes. *(D):* A close-up of the area in brackets is shown in *(C)*. The central portion shows a lymphoid-type follicle surrounded by lymphocytes/plasmacytes. Movat stain, X40 *(B)*; hematoxylin/eosin stain, X40 *(C)* and X400 *(D)*.

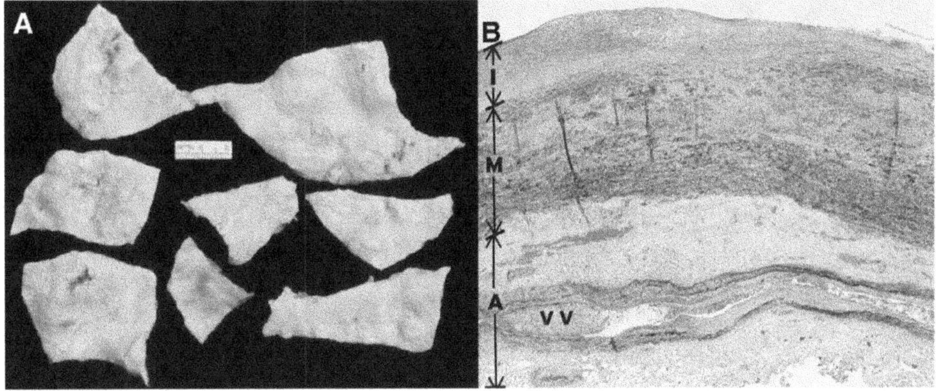

Fig. 8. Patient #22. *(A):* Fragments of the excised tubular portion of ascending aorta. Every square millimeter of the intimal surface is abnormal. *(B):* Photomicrograph of a portion of aorta. The intima (I) is thickened by fibrous tissue, there is severe loss of elastic fibers in the media (M), and there is severe scarring of the adventitia (A), which contains a vasa vasorum (VV), the wall of which is thickened and the lumen narrowed. Movat stain, X40 *(B)*.

## Disclosures

The authors have no conflicts of interest to disclose.

1. Roberts WC, Bose R, Ko JM, Henry AC, Hamman BL. Identifying cardiovascular syphilis at operation. *Am J Cardiol* 2009;104(11):1588–1594.
2. Roberts WC, Lensing FD, Kourlis H Jr, Ko JM, Newberry JW, Smerud MJ, Burton EC, Hebeler RF Jr. Full blown cardiovascular syphilis with aneurysm of the innominate artery. *Am J Cardiol* 2009;104(11):1595–1600.
3. Roberts WC, Ko JM, Vowels TJ. Natural history of syphilitic aortitis. *Am J Cardiol* 2009;104(11):1578–1587.
4. Roberts WC, Barbin CM, Weissenborn MR, Ko JM. Electrocardiographic total 12-lead QRS voltage in patients having operative resection of syphilitic aortic aneurysm. *Am J Cardiol* 2015;116 (6):973–976.

5. Roberts WC, Barbin CM, Weissenborn MR, Ko JM, Henry AC. Syphilis as a cause of thoracic aortic aneurysm. *Am J Cardiol* 2015;116(8):1298–1303.

6. Barbin CM, Weissenborn MR, Ko JM, Guileyardo JE, Roberts WC. Computed tomographic and morphologic features of syphilis of the aorta. *Am J Cardiol* 2015;116(8):1311–1314.

7. Sundt TM 3rd, Roberts WC. Thoralf Mauritz Sundt III, MD: A conversation with the editor. *Am J Cardiol* 2017;119(1):156–168.

8. Sprecher DL, Schaefer EJ, Kent KM, Gregg RE, Zech LA, Hoeg JM, Mcmanus B, Roberts WC, Brewer HB. Cardiovascular features of homozygous familial hypercholesterolemia: analysis of 16 patients. *Am J Cardiol* 1984;54:20–30.

9. Roberts WC, Won VS, Weissenborn MR, Khalid A, Lima B. Massive diffuse calcification of the ascending aorta in heterozygous familial hypercholesterolemia. *Am J Cardiol* 2016:1381–1385.

# Syphilitic aortitis: still a current common cause of aneurysm of the tubular portion of ascending aorta

William C. Roberts [a, b, *], Alastair J. Moore [c], Charles S. Roberts [d]

[a] Baylor Scott & White Heart and Vascular Institute, Baylor University Medical Center, Dallas, TX, USA
[b] Department of Internal Medicine (Cardiology Division) and Pathology, Baylor University Medical Center, Dallas, TX, USA
[c] Department of Radiology Baylor University Medical Center, Dallas, TX, USA
[d] Department of Cardiac Surgery, Baylor University Medical Center, Dallas, TX, USA

## ARTICLE INFO

Article history:
Received 24 September 2019
Received in revised form
16 October 2019
Accepted 22 October 2019

Keywords:
Aortic syphilis
Aortitis
Aortic aneurysm
Aortic regurgitation

## ABSTRACT

Aortic syphilis today is infrequently diagnosed clinically. Described herein are findings in 5 women who had resection of a fusiform aneurysm of the tubular portion of ascending aorta, and examination of the wall of the aneurysm disclosed classic features of aortic syphilis. The 5 patients were among 36 who had ascending aortic operations at Baylor University Medical Center in Dallas in 2018 and early 2019. Syphilitic aneurysm in each spared the sinus portion and involved diffusely the tubular portion of ascending aorta, beginning at the sinotubular junction. The aneurysmal wall was thicker than normal because of thickening of both intima and adventitia. The latter contained foci of lymphocytes and plasmacytes and thickened and narrowed vasa vasora. The media was disrupted by fibrous scars, which weakened the integrity of the aorta. Aortitis of the tubular portion of ascending aorta in syphilis is a diffuse process, but often is mistakenly called "atherosclerosis" which, when present in this portion of aorta, can be extensive but is focal. Aortic syphilis is important to diagnose so that patients can receive antibiotic therapy to delay, prevent, or treat neurosyphilis, a common accompaniment of aortic syphilis.

© 2019 Elsevier Inc. All rights reserved.

## 1. Introduction

In recent years, several articles have appeared describing classic gross and histologic features of syphilis of the aorta and they have emphasized its role as a common cause of fusiform and saccular aneurysms of the ascending aorta [1–6]. Despite these publications, patients with chronic aneurysms of the tubular position of ascending aorta continue to be treated without consideration that the aneurysm may be the result of syphilis: a serologic test for syphilis is not performed; the resected aorta submitted to surgical pathology is not diagnosed as aortic syphilis, and most of these patients never receive appropriate antibiotic therapy to delay, prevent, or treat the occurrence of neurological syphilis. This report simply adds to previous ones to emphasize that aortic syphilis is indeed back, needs to be properly diagnosed, and requires appropriate antibiotic therapy.

* Corresponding author. Baylor Scott & White Heart and Vascular Institute, 621 N. Hall Street, Suite H-030, Dallas, TX, 75226, USA. Fax: (214) 820-7533.
E-mail address: William.Roberts1@bswhealth.org (W.C. Roberts).

## 2. Materials and methods

This report describes pertinent clinical and morphologic findings in five women, who underwent operative resection of a fusiform aneurysm of the tubular portion of ascending aorta at Baylor University Medical Center (BUMC) during 2018 and the first 2 months of 2019, and histologic study of the aneurysmal wall showed classic features of aortic syphilis. These five patients were among 43 patients who underwent resection of all or a portion of the tubular portion of ascending aorta at BUMC in 2018 and early

**Table 1**
Resection of ascending aortic aneurysm at the Baylor University Medical Center (January 2018–February 2019) (14 months)

| Causes | Number of cases |
|---|---|
| Aortic dissection | 23 (58%) |
| Associated with a unicuspid or bicuspid aortic valve | 9 (22%) |
| Associated with purely regurgitant tricuspid aortic valve secondary to probable systemic hypertension (2 patients) or sinus of Valsalva aneurysm (1 patient) | 3 (8%) |
| Syphilis | 5 (12%) |
| Total | 40 |

**Table 2**
Clinical and morphologic features in each of the 5 women with aortic syphilis

| Variable | Case #1 | Case #2 | Case #3 | Case #4 | Case #5 |
| --- | --- | --- | --- | --- | --- |
| Age (years) at operation | 68 | 68 | 70 | 71 | 76 |
| Symptoms | None | DOE[a] | DOE[a] | DOE[b] | None |
| Diameter, ascending aorta (cm) | 6.0 | 5.5 | 5.1 | 6.3 | 6.0 |
| Body mass index (kg/m$^2$) | 24 | 25 | 29 | 29 | 30 |
| LV cavity size | Normal | Normal | Normal | Normal | Normal |
| LV ejection fraction (%) | 50 | 60 | 60 | 65 | 35 |
| Aortic regurgitation | Trace | 0 | 0 | Mild | Moderate |
| Total 12-lead QRS voltage (mm) | 98 | 92 | 169 | 99 | 202 |
| Diabetes mellitus | 0 | 0 | 0 | 0 | + |
| Smoker | ++ | ++[b] | ++ | +++[b] | 0 |
| Blood pressure (mm Hg) | 143/73 (D) | 105/65 (I) | 175/63 (D) | 110/50 (I) | 190/80 (I) |
| Weight (g) resected aorta | 25 | 10 | 13 | 16 | 18 |
| Total cholesterol (mg/dL) | 167 | 214 | 186 | – | 173 |
| LDL cholesterol (mg/dL) | 96 | 115 | 68 | – | 121 |
| Coronary arteries by angiogram | Normal | Minor↓ | Normal | Normal | Normal |
| Aortic valve surgery | None | None | None | Replaced | Resuspended |

Abbreviations: D = direct (at cardiac catheterization); DOE = dyspnea on exertion; I = indirect (blood pressure cuff); LDL = low-density lipoprotein; LV = left ventricular.
[a] Etiology unclear.
[b] Severe chronic obstructive pulmonary disease.

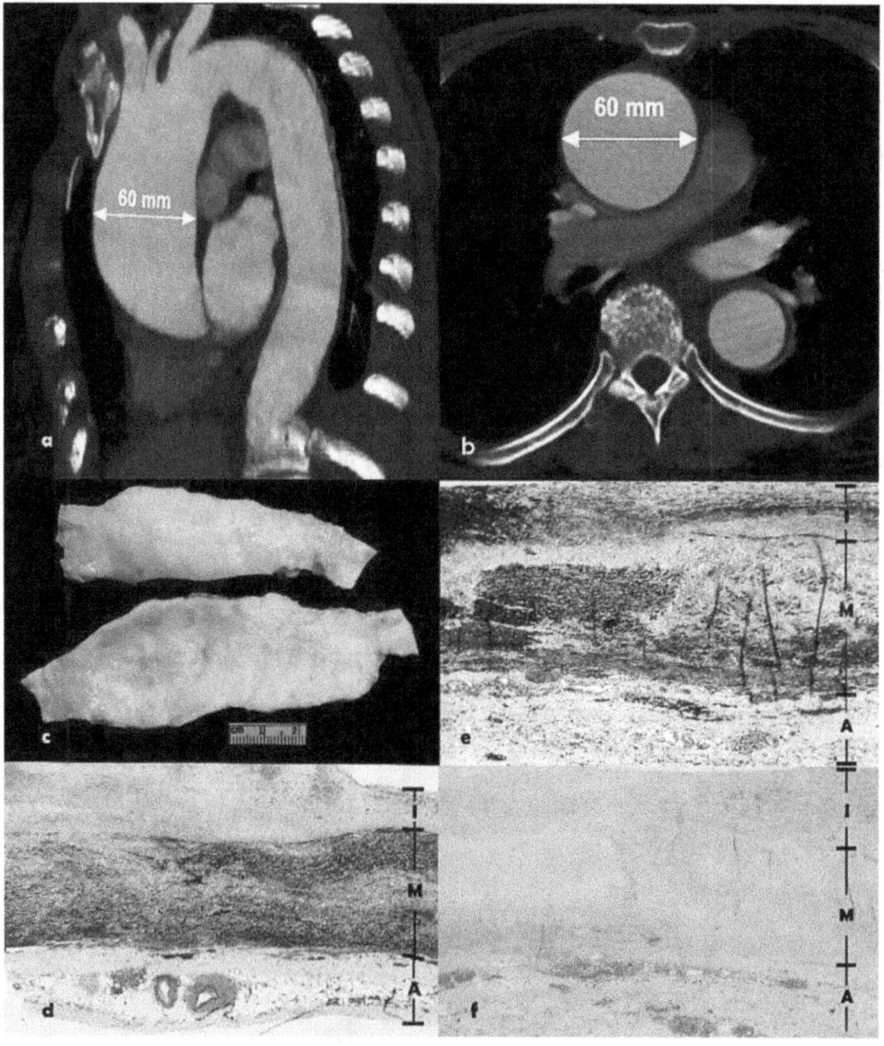


**Fig. 1.** (Case #1, Table 2). Shown here are sagittal maximum intensity projection (MIP) and axial multiplanar reformat (MPR) computed tomography angiography (CTA) images (a, b) and photographs (gross and microscopic) of the aorta (c–f). (a). Considerable dilatation of the tubular portion of ascending aorta is present and the sinus portion is not dilated. (c) The resected aorta. There is 100% abnormality of the intimal surface, a clue to the diagnosis of syphilitic aortitis. (d) Photomicrograph of the wall of the aorta. It is divided into intima (I), media (M), and adventitia (A). The intima is thickened, mainly by fibrous tissue including elastic fibers, there is considerable loss of elastic fibers in the media and the adventitia is thickened by fibrous tissue. The vasa vasora in the adventitia are thickened. (e) Another portion of ascending aorta again with thickened intima, loss of elastic fibers in the media, and thickened adventitia. (f) Collections of lymphocytes and plasma cells in the adventitia. Movat stains (d and e) X 40, hematoxylin and eosin stain (f) X 100.

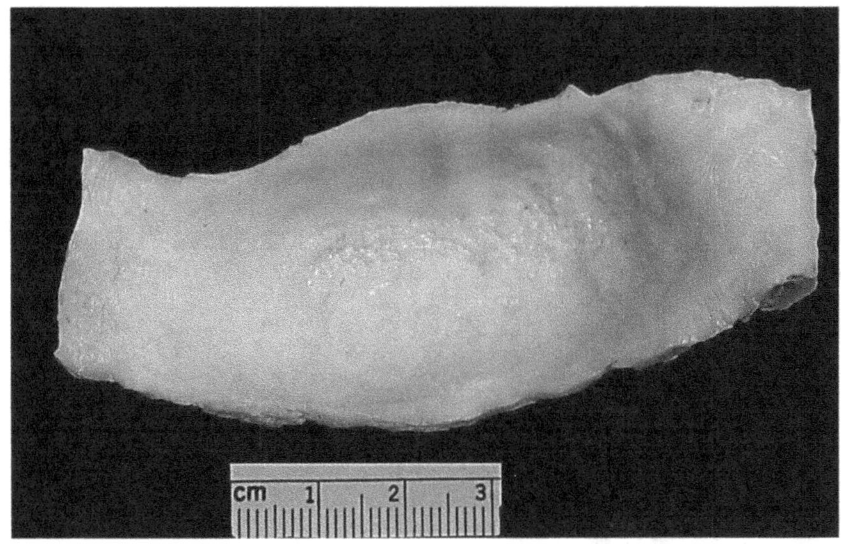

**Fig. 2.** (Case #2, Table 2). Opened aorta showing 100% intimal surface abnormality typical of aortic syphilis.

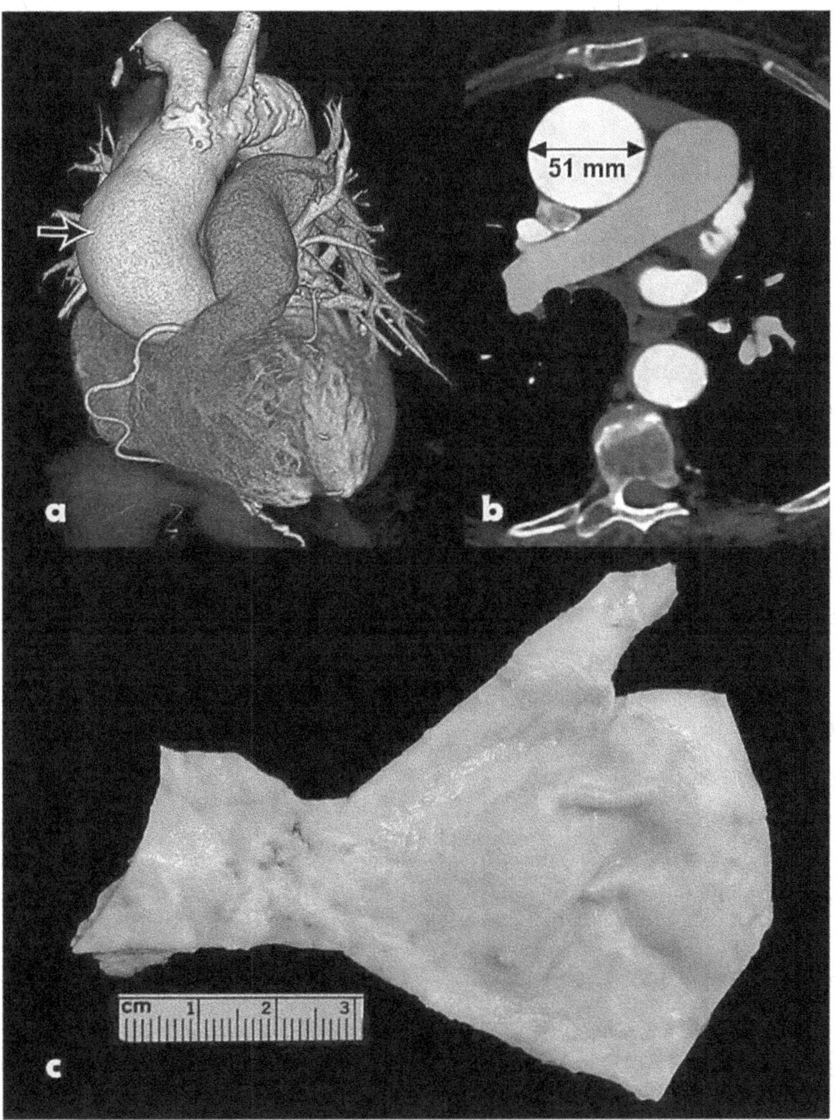


**Fig. 3.** (Case #3, Table 2.). (a) Three-dimensional surface projection derived from computed tomography angiography (CTA) images of the great arteries and heart. The tubular portion of ascending aorta is dilated, and the sinus portion is not. (b) An axial CTA image of the dilated ascending aorta. (c) View of the excised tubular potion of ascending aorta. Every square mm is abnormal.

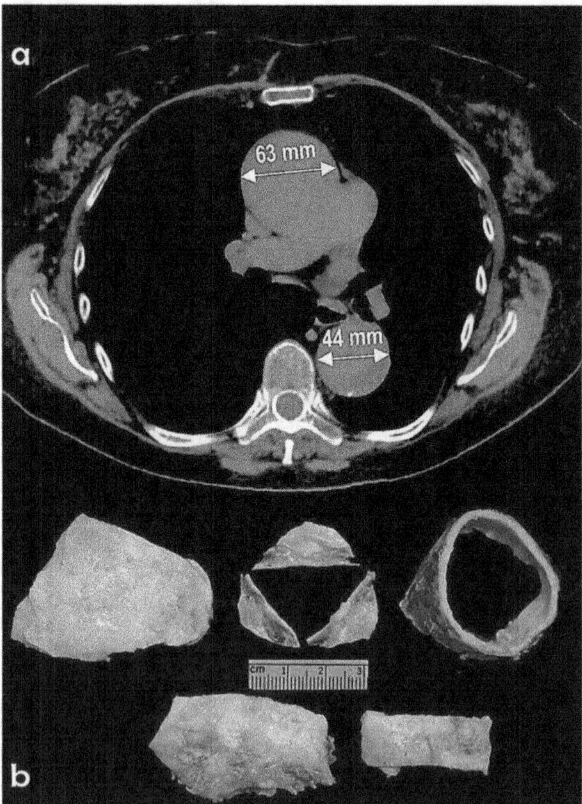

**Fig. 4.** (Case #4, Table 2.). (a) A noncontrast axial computed tomography (CT) image of the dilated tubular portion of ascending aorta. (b) Four fragments of the operatively excised ascending aorta. The intima in each is 100% abnormal. This patient had excision of the tricuspid aortic valve, the free margins of which are mildly thickened centrally by fibrous tissue.

2019 (Table 1). The aneurysmal walls were submitted to surgical pathology where they were examined and described, sections cut, and stained by both hematoxylin and eosin and Movat methods, and examined by examined by one of the authors (WCR).

## 3. Results

Pertinent findings in the 5 patients are tabulated in Table 2. All 5 were white women aged 67–76 years at the time of the aneurysmal resection. Two of the 5 patients were asymptomatic, and dilatation of the ascending aorta was discovered by incidental chest radiograph; 2 patients (#2 and #3, Table 2) had exertional dyspnea that prompted an extensive workup; another had chronic obstructive pulmonary disease (Her dyspnea was likely the result of the pulmonary disease.). In each patient, the aortic aneurysm began at the sinotubular junction and ended just caudal to the origin of the brachiocephalic artery (Figs. 1–5). In all 5 patients, the maximal transverse diameter by computed tomography ranged from 5.1 to 6.3 cm, the diameter of the sinus portion of aorta was normal, the left ventricular cavity was of normal size, and the aortic valve was tricuspid. Trace to moderate aortic regurgitation occurred in 3 of the 5 patients. The left ventricular ejection fraction was normal in 4 and low (35%) in 1 patient. The peak systolic systemic arterial pressures were elevated (>140 mmHg) in 3 patients and the pulse pressures were widened (≥60 mmHg) in 4 patients. Angiogram in all 5 patients showed normal or nearly normal epicardial coronary arteries. The body mass indexes ranged from 24 to 30 kg/m$^2$. Total 12-lead QRS voltage [7,8] was <100 mm in 3 patients and 169 and 202 in the other 2 patients, respectively[7]. All 5 patients had uncomplicated postoperative courses except for the occurrence of atrial fibrillation, only one of whom (patient #2, Table 1) had the arrhythmias preoperatively.

In each patient, the ascending aorta was replaced by a graft. At gross examination of the aneurysm in all 5 patients, the intimal surface was diffusely abnormal, and its wall was thickened. Histologic examination disclosed thickened intima (mainly by fibrous tissue with or without focal lipid and calcific deposits), focal loss of medial elastic fibers, and adventitia thickened by fibrous tissue that contained foci of lymphocytes and plasmacytes and thickened vasa vasora (Figs. 1–5), findings characteristic of syphilitic aortitis.

## 4. Discussion

Described herein are clinical, radiographic, and morphologic findings in 5 women whose dilated tubular portion of aorta was resected and found to be characteristic of aortic syphilis. The morphologic findings in these 5 patients, to our knowledge, have not been observed in any condition other than syphilis. Although the intimal abnormality may suggest atherosclerosis, when present in the ascending aorta, the atherosclerotic process is always focal (except in patients with homozygous familial hypercholesterolemia [9,10]), its media is usually spared, and its adventitia neither is thickened by fibrous tissue nor contains collections of inflammatory cells (lymphocytes and plasmacytes) (Table 3).

Atherosclerosis can occur in any portion of the aorta although the syphilitic process spares the sinus portion of aorta and usually, with some exceptions, does not affect the arch or descending thoracic portions of aorta. Despite reports to the contrary [11], syphilis never affects the abdominal aorta because there are no vasa vasora in that portion of aorta. Occasionally in aortic syphilis, one or more saccular aneurysms are present in the thoracic aorta and/or arch arteries, sometimes arising from the fusiform aneurysm, and thrombus is present within the saccular aneurysm. The result of these anatomic changes is that the wall of the aorta is thicker than normal, but functionally it is weaker than normal (i.e., it dilates) presumably because the integrity of the media has been disrupted by focal scars. The "strength" of the aorta, like all arteries, appears to be dependent on the integrity of the media.

Because syphilis is infrequently considered clinically, radiologically, or at operation as the cause of an aneurysm involving the tubular portion of ascending aorta, we suggest that all such patients have proper serologic tests for syphilis [12], even though a negative result does not necessarily mean the absence of aortic syphilis. The characteristic gross and histologic features in the operatively resected aortas, indicative of syphilitic aortitis, support the position that appropriate antibiotics should be administered to delay or prevent the occurrence of neurosyphilis, a frequent accompaniment of aortic syphilis.

It is recognized that panaortitis has causes other than syphilis, but its location is different from aortic syphilis. Ankylosing spondylitis in the aorta is similar to syphilis histologically but its involvement of the aorta is limited to the aortic valve commissures and the aorta for about a centimeter just cephalad to the sinotubular junction [13]. In addition, ankylosing spondylitis involves the wall of the aorta in the sinus portion and extends into the anterior mitral leaflet and membranous ventricular septum. Aortic syphilis, in contrast, never extends into the wall of aorta bordering the sinuses of Valsalva or caudal to the aortic valve. The aortic valve cusps are not involved in syphilis.

Panaortitis is seen, of course, in several nonsyphilitic conditions which involve not just the aorta but many of the branches arising from the aorta [14–17]. Temporal arteritis mainly involves, of course, the temporal arteries and commonly also causes severe thickening of both the intima and adventitia [17]. Giant cells occur commonly in this condition as well as numerous inflammatory cells. Syphilis never involves the temporal arteries. Giant cell

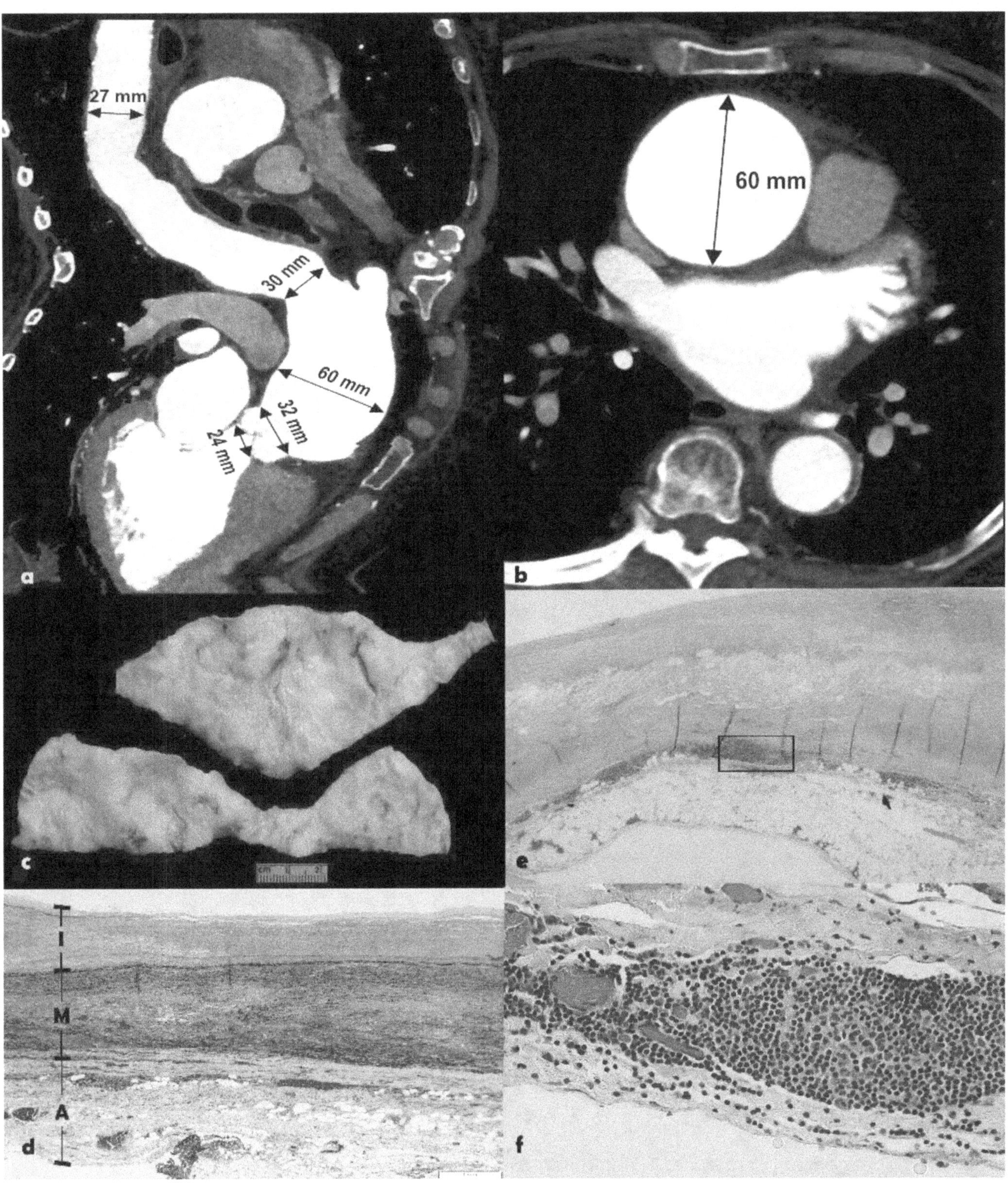

**Fig. 5.** (Case #5, Table 2.). (a) Curved multiplanar reformat (cMPR) derived from computed tomography angiography (CTA) images of the thoracic aorta; the tubular portion of ascending aorta is quite dilated, and the sinus portion of ascending aorta is not dilated; (b) Axial CTA image of the tubular portion of dilated ascending aorta; (c) Portion of ascending aorta excised. The intima is 100% abnormal; (d) Movat-stained section of aorta. The intima is thickened, there is considerable loss of medial elastic fibers in the media , and the adventitia is thickened; (e) A hematoxylin and eosin stain of a portion of aorta showing collections of lymphocytes and plasma cells in the adventitia, and (f) Close-up of these cells shown in the rectangle of (e) Movat stain X 40 (d), hematoxylin and eosin stain X 40 (e), and X 400 (f).

**Table 3**
Morphologic differences between aortic syphilis and atherosclerosis

| Disease | Wall of ascending aorta | | |
|---|---|---|---|
| | Intima | Media | Adventitia |
| Atherosclerosis | + (focal) | 0 | 0 |
| Syphilis | + (diffuse) | + (scarred) | + (thickened) (inflammatory cells) (abnormal vasa vasora) |

+ = abnormal; 0 = normal.

aortitis usually also involves not only the aorta but many of its branches. Giant cells are uncommon in the aortic wall in patients with syphilis and it is also associated with thickening of the walls of the vasa vasora, something not common in giant cell aortitis. Idiopathic aortitis not only involves the aorta but also arteries arising from the aorta including the coronary [14–16]. Involvement of the heart itself, not uncommon in nonsyphilitic aortitis, does not occur in syphilis, which may narrow the ostium of one or both coronary ostia, but this is a consequence of its involvement of the aorta, not the coronary arteries directly. Nearly all of the idiopathic aortitis group contains giant cells among the inflammatory infiltrates. Panaortitis secondary to rheumatic or rheumatoid disease is extremely rare and morphologically different from aortic syphilis [18]. Systemic lupus erythematosus has not been seen by us despite study of numerous cases at autopsy [19–21].

The positive feature of the present study is that investigators with extensive previous experience with aortic syphilis produced it. Its major deficiency is that none of the 5 patients had preoperative serologic tests for syphilis, which, however, may or may not be positive or reactive in patients with aortic syphilis. Other tests to rule out other forms of panaortitis were not performed.

## Funding

This research did not receive any specific grant from funding agencies in the public, commercial, or not-for-profit sectors.

## Conflicts of interest

None.

## Acknowledgments

The authors would like to thank Saba Ilyas for her photographic talents.

## References

[1] Roberts WC, Ko JM, Vowels TJ. Natural history of syphilitic aortitis. Am J Cardiol 2009;104:1578–87.

[2] Roberts WC, Bose R, Ko JM, Henry AC, Hamman BL. Identifying cardiovascular syphilis at operation. Am J Cardiol 2009;104:1588–94.

[3] Roberts WC, Lensing FD, Kourlis Jr H, Ko JM, Newberry JW, Smerud MJ, et al. Full blown cardiovascular syphilis with aneurysm of the innominate artery. Am J Cardiol 2009;104:1595–600.

[4] Roberts WC, Barbin CM, Weissenborn MR, Ko JM, Henry AC. Syphilis as a cause of thoracic aortic aneurysm. Am J Cardiol 2015;116(8):1298–303.

[5] Barbin CM, Weissenborn MR, Ko JM, Guileyardo JE, Roberts WC. Computed tomographic and morphologic features of syphilis of the aorta. Am J Cardiol 2015;116:1311–4.

[6] Roberts WC, Kondapalli N. Operative recognition of syphilis of the aorta. Am J Cardiol 2018;122(5):898–904.

[7] Roberts WC, Filardo G, Ko JM, Siegel RJ, Dollar AL, Ross EM, et al. Comparison of total 12-lead QRS voltage in a variety of cardiac conditions and its usefulness in predicting increased cardiac mass. Am J Cardiol 2013;112(6):904–9.

[8] Roberts WC, Barbin CM, Weissenborn MR, Ko JM. Electrocardiographic total 12-lead QRS voltage in patients having operative resection of syphilitic aortic aneurysm. Am J Cardiol 2015;116:973–6.

[9] Sprecher DL, Schaefer EJ, Kent KM, Gregg RE, Zech LA, Hoeg JM, et al. Cardiovascular features of homozygous familial hypercholesterolemia. Analysis of 16 patients. Am J Cardiol 1984;54:20–30.

[10] Kragel AH, Roberts WC. Composition of atherosclerotic plaques in the coronary arteries in homozygous familial hypercholesterolemia. Am Heart J 1991;121:210–1.

[11] Marconato R, Inzaghi A, Cantoni GM, Zappa M, Longo T. Syphilitic aneurysm of the abdominal aorta: report of two cases. Eur J Vasc Surg 1988;2(3):199–203.

[12] Cantor AG, Pappas M, Daegas M, Nelson HD. Screening for syphilis. Updated evidence report and systemic review for the U.S. Preventive Services Task Force. J Am Med Assoc 2016;315:2328–37.

[13] Bulkley BH, Roberts WC. Ankylosing spondylitis and aortic regurgitation: description of the characteristic cardiovascular lesion from study of eight necropsy patients. Circulation 1973;48:1014–27.

[14] Roberts WC, Wibin EA. Idiopathic panaortitis, supraaortic arteritis, granulomatous myocarditis and pericarditis. A cause of pulseless disease and possibly left ventricular aneurysm in the African. Am J Med 1966;41:453–61.

[15] Roberts WC, MacGregor RR, DeBlanc HJ, Beiser GD, Wolff SM. The prepulseless phase of pulseless disease, or pulseless disease with pulses. A newly recognized cause of cardiac disease, monoclonal gammopathy and "fever of unknown origin". Am J Med 1969;46:313–24.

[16] Honig HS, Weintraub AM, Gomes MN, Hufnagel CA, Roberts WC. Severe aortic regurgitation secondary to idiopathic aortitis. Am J Med 1977;63:623–33.

[17] Roberts WC, Zafar S, Ko JM. Morphological features of temporal arteritis. Proc (Bayl Univ Med Cent) 2013;26:109–15.

[18] Carpenter DF, Golden A, Roberts WC. Quadrivalvular rheumatoid heart disease associated with left bundle branch block. Am J Med 1967;43:922–9.

[19] Bulkley BH, Roberts WC. The heart in systemic lupus erythematosus and the changes induced in it by corticosteroid therapy: a study of 36 necropsy patients. Am J Med 1975;58:243–64.

[20] Haider YS, Roberts WC. Coronary arterial disease in systemic lupus erythematosus: quantification of degrees of narrowing in 22 necropsy patients (21 women) aged 16 to 37 years. Am J Med 1981;70:775–81.

[21] Roberts WC, High ST. The heart in systemic lupus erythematosus. Curr Probl Cardiol 1999;24(#1):1–56.

# Combined Cardiovascular Syphilis and Aortic Valve Stenosis (Due to a Congenitally Unicuspid Valve)

Madiha Makhdumi, MBBS, MPH[a], and William C. Roberts, MD[a,b,*]

**Described herein is a 53-year-old man who underwent resection of a fusiform aneurysm of the ascending aorta, and excision of a congenitally malformed stenotic unicuspid aortic valve. Examination of the wall of the aortic aneurysm disclosed classic features of syphilis. Although some degree of pure aortic regurgitation is common in patients with aortic syphilis, the presence of associated aortic valve stenosis, such as occurred in this patient, has been mentioned in only 4 previous publications, none of which included morphologic examination of the ascending aorta or aortic valve. © 2022 Elsevier Inc. All rights reserved. (Am J Cardiol 2022;172:144−145)**

It is well known that aortic syphilis is often associated with chronic aortic regurgitation, usually of rather mild degree. If aortic syphilis occurs in a patient with aortic valve stenosis, the cause of the valve condition is unrelated to the syphilis. Recently, we examined an operatively-excised stenotic aortic valve which was congenitally abnor-

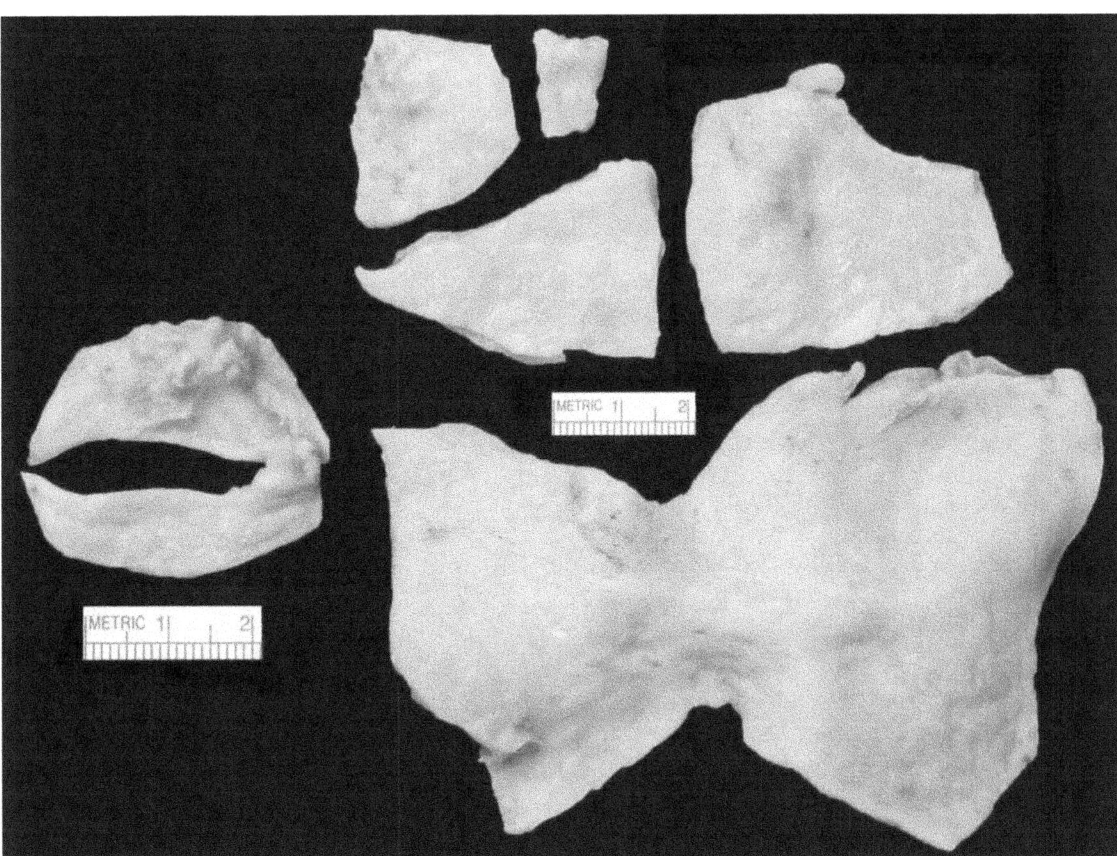



Figure 1. View of the operatively excised unicuspid, unicommisural valve and the excised tubular portion of the ascending aorta (5.5 cm in diameter) in the patient described. The unicuspid valve has focal calcific deposits. One true commissure is present, and the orifice has a linear appearance similar to an exclamation point. The commissure opposite the true commissure is calcified. Fragments of the ascending aorta resected at operation are shown on the right. The intimal surface is granular in appearance and some portions have a grayish tint. The wall of the aorta is much thicker than normal.

[a]From the Baylor Heart and Vascular Institute; and [b]the Departments of Internal Medicine and Pathology, Baylor University Medical Center, Dallas, Texas. Manuscript received February 1, 2022; revised manuscript received and accepted February 15, 2022.

*Corresponding Author: William C. Roberts, MD, Baylor Scott & White Heart and Vascular Institute, Baylor University Medical Center, 621 N. Hall Street, Suite H-030, Dallas, Texas 75226, (214) 820-7911 Phone, (214) 820-7533 Fax

*E-mail address:* william.roberts1@bswhealth.org (W.C. Roberts).

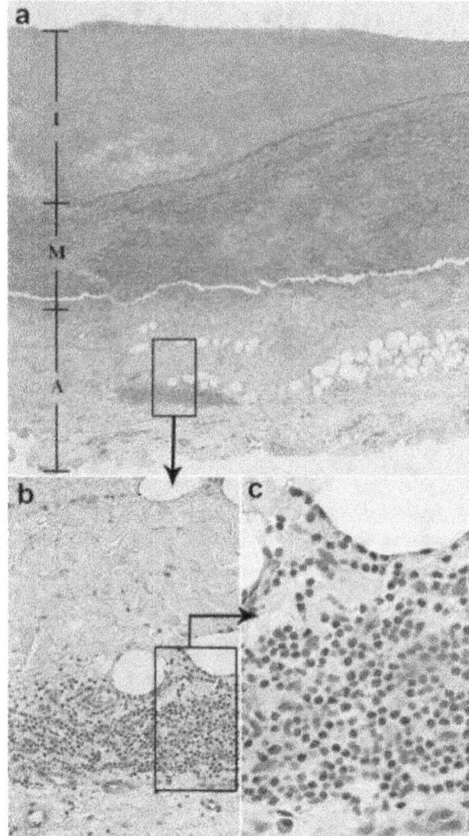

Figure 2. Portions of aorta in the patient described. a, Photomicrograph of a portion of ascending aorta. The intima (I) and adventitia (A) are thickened, mainly by fibrous tissue. The adventitia contains large collections of lymphocytes and plasma cells. The media (M) is not thickened but focally many elastic fibers are replaced by fibrous tissue. b, A closer view of the collection of cells bracketed. in a. c, An even closer view of the collection of lymphocytes and plasma cells bracketed in b. Movat stains X 40(a), X 400(b), X 1000(c).

mal and a resected ascending aorta with classic features of aortic syphilis. Such an occurrence we have not encountered previously. Search of PubMed disclosed 4 such cases, none of which documented morphologically the presence of aortic syphilis.[1-4]

## Case Study

A 53-year-old traveling salesman, who was born in November 1964, was in his usual health until approximately June 2017 when he sought medical care for what proved to be atrial tachycardia and an ablation procedure was done. At that time, imaging studies showed his ascending aorta to be dilated (5.5 cm). During the next year he developed periodic episodes of substernal chest discomfort relieved by nitroglycerin. Echocardiogram showed the mean gradient between left ventricle and aorta to be 10 mmHg and the peak gradient to be 20 mmHg. Angiogram showed all epicardial coronary arteries to be normal. The left ventricular cavity was of nor-

mal size and its ejection fraction was about 60%. In July 2018, both the aortic valve and ascending aorta were replaced (Bio-Bentall procedure): the valve was replaced with a 29-mm Trifecta bioprosthesis. His postoperative course was uncomplicated. When seen in July 2019 he had no symptoms attributable to his heart and aorta.

The operatively excised aortic valve and the excised ascending aorta is shown in figure 1 and histologic features of the aorta in figure 2. The slides of the aorta were stained for IgG4 and it was negative (very few IgG4 cells were positive).

## Comments

As far as we can determine, the heretofore described patient is the first to be reported with a congenitally malformed mildly stenotic aortic valve associated with classic morphologic features of aortic syphilis. These features include thickening of the aortic intima by fibrous tissue with or without calcific deposits, marked focal loss of elastic fibers in the media with replacement by fibrous tissue, and marked thickening of the adventitia which contains thickened vasa vasora with narrowed lumens and focal collections of mononuclear cells (lymphocytes and plasmacytes).[5-8]

A limitation of this report is the absence of the performance of the rapid plasma reagin and fluorescent treponemal antibody tests, both of which may be negative or nonreactive in the presence of aortic syphilis.

## Declaration of interests

The authors declare that they have no known competing financial interests or personal relationships that could have appeared to influence the work reported in this paper.


1. Richter AB. Treponema pallidum in syphilitic aortic valvulitis of a congenitally bicuspid valve with subaortic stenosis: report of a case. *Am J Pathol* 1936;12:129–140.
2. Gunther L, Van OT, Kaplan L. Calcareous nodular stenosis of the aortic valve with syphilitic aortitis and aneurysm. *Ann West Med Surg* 1949;3:287–294.
3. Krylov AA, Sapego AV, Onishchenko KF. Izolirovannyĭ kal'tsifitsirovannyĭ klapannyĭ stenoz aorty pri tretichnom sifilise [Isolated calcified aortic valve stenosis in tertiary syphilis]. *Revmatologiia (Mosk)* 1990;4:74–75.
4. Sorokin A, Weich H, Doubell A, Moolman JA. Bilateral ostial coronary stenosis and rheumatic aortic valve stenosis. *Acute Card Care* 2006;8:113–115.
5. Roberts WC, Bose R, Ko JM, Henry AC, Hamman BL. Identifying cardiovascular syphilis at operation. *Am J Cardiol* 2009;104:1588–1594.
6. Roberts WC, Ko JM, Vowels TJ. Natural history of syphilitic aortitis. *Am J Cardiol* 2009;104:1578–1587.
7. Roberts WC, Barbin CM, Weissenborn MR, Ko JM, Henry AC. Syphilis as a cause of thoracic aortic aneurysm. *Am J Cardiol* 2015;116:1298–1303.
8. Roberts WC, Moore AJ, Roberts CS. Syphilitic aortitis: still a current common cause of aneurysm of the tubular portion of ascending aorta. *Cardiovasc Pathol* 2020;46:107175.

# Combined Cardiovascular Syphilis and Type A Acute Aortic Dissection

William C. Roberts, MD[a,b,c,*], and Charles S. Roberts, MD[a,d]

**The occurrence of acute aortic dissection with the initiating tear in the ascending aorta superimposed on cardiovascular syphilis is an exceedingly rare occurrence. Such was the case, however, in a recently seen patient who presented with typical features of acute dissection (type A). Operative repair yielded the entire ascending aorta to examine both grossly and histologically and classic features of both conditions were observed.** © 2021 Elsevier Inc. All rights reserved. (Am J Cardiol 2022;168:159−162)

## Introduction

A number of authors for many decades have listed cardiovascular syphilis as a potential predisposing factor for aortic dissection. We have been hesitant to accept this relationship because cardiovascular syphilis begins in the adventitia, causes severe focal loss of medial elastic fibers, replacing them with scar tissue, and considerable thickening of the intima. Aortic dissection, in contrast, is a medial disease associated with none or only minimal loss of its elastic fibers and is unassociated with thickening of either the adventitia or intima. Recently, we encountered for the first time a patient who underwent resection of the ascending aorta because of a large intimal-medial tear leading to dissection of the ascending aorta and beyond and associated with classic morphologic features of cardiovascular syphilis.

## Case Study

A 78-year-old man with known cerebral aneurysm and infarction was in his usual state of health until about one hour before admission to Baylor University Medical Center (BUMC) when while sitting watching television he suddenly passed out and when awakening noted severe right arm and chest pain and nausea. Emergency medical service brought him to the hospital. At examination, his blood pressure was 115 / 70 mm Hg. A precordial murmur was absent. The left-sided radial pulses were absent. His heart rate was 65 beats / minute. Not long after arriving to BUMC he had cardiac arrest. Cardiac resuscitation was initiated. Orotracheal intubation was carried out. Circulation was restored. A nasogastric tube was inserted. An electrocardiogram was negative for myocardial ischemia. Computed thoracic angiogram disclosed a type A acute aortic dissection (Figure 1). There was delayed filling of the common carotid arteries and the right subclavian artery. At operation, a large tear was present just cephalad to the sino-tubular junction, the ascending aorta was

From the [a]Baylor Scott & White Heart and Vascular Institute, the Departments of [b]Internal Medicine, [c]Pathology, and [d]Cardiac and Thoracic Surgery, Baylor University Medical Center, Baylor Scott & White Health, Dallas, Texas. Manuscript received October 4, 2021; revised manuscript received and accepted October 29, 2021.

*Corresponding Author: William C. Roberts, MD, Baylor Scott & White Heart and Vascular Institute, 621 N. Hall Street, Suite H-030, Dallas, Texas 75226, (214) 820-7911 Office, (214) 820-7533 Fax

*E-mail address:* william.roberts1@bswhealth.org (W.C. Roberts).

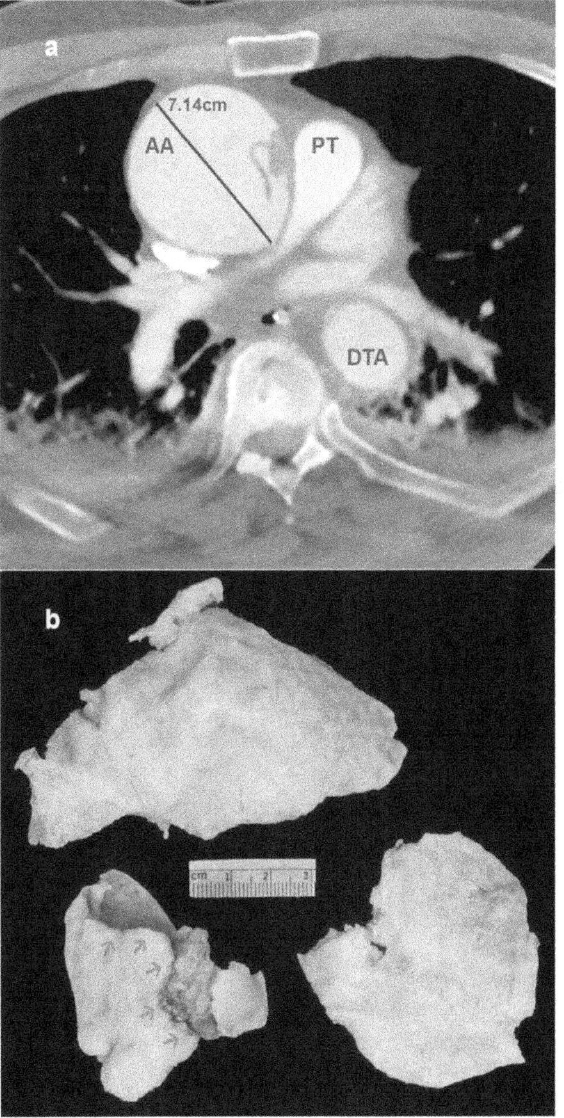


Figure 1. Shown here is the computer tomographic image of the heart and great arteries before the ascending aorta (AA) was resected. a The ascending aorta is hugely dilated, and it narrows a bit the adjacent pulmonary trunk (PT). The ascending aorta is much larger than the descending thoracic aorta (DTA). b Fragments of aorta resected by the surgeon (CSR). There is diffuse abnormality of the aortic intima -every square mm abnormal. The dissection tear is present in the lower left portion of this figure (arrows).

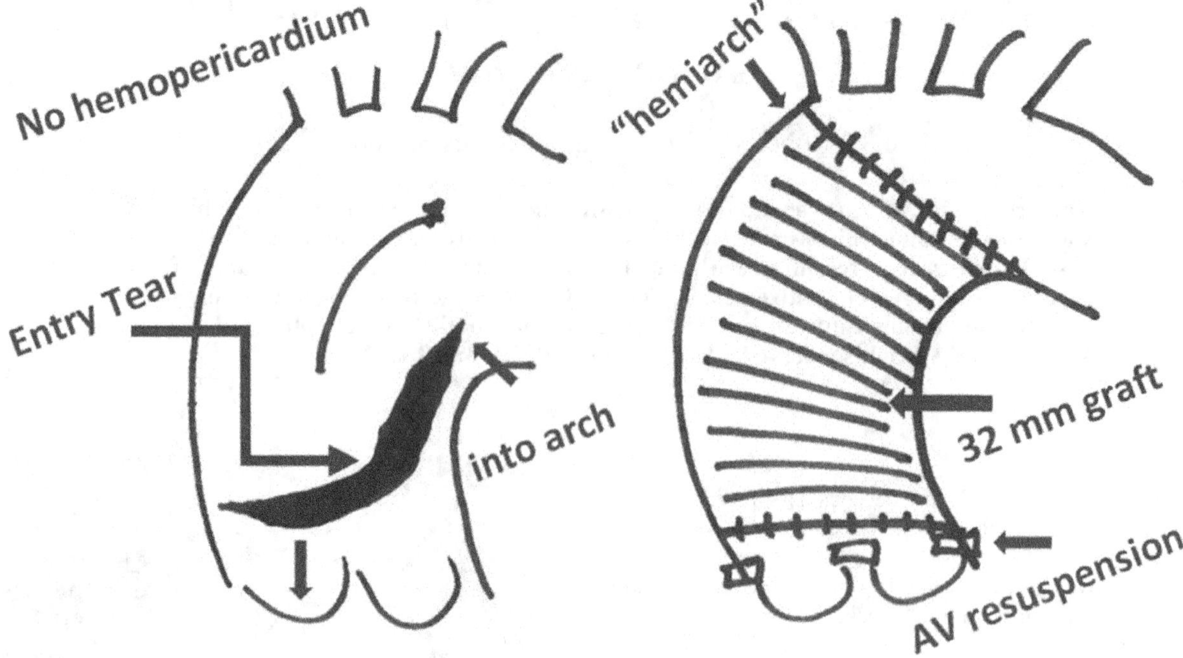


Figure 2.  An illustration depicting the ascending aortic entry tear and the subsequent graft replacement.

resected, and the 3 aortic cusps were resuspended at their commissures (Figure 2.)

The ascending aorta was removed in 3 pieces, one of which contained a large intimal-medial tear that initiated the acute medial dissection (Figures 1 and 2). The intimal surface was diffusely abnormal. Histologically, (Figure 3) the adventitia was thickened by fibrosis tissue that contained numerous focal collections of plasmacytes and lymphocytes. Additionally, scattered in other areas of the adventitia were many eosinophils. The vasa vasora in the adventitia had thickened walls and narrowed lumens. The dissection was in the very outer media and often between the external elastic membrane and the outer media. There was massive loss of medial elastic fibers. The intima was thickened, mainly by fibrous tissue, and also by focal calcific deposits.

**Discussion**

In the last 60 years we have studied about 200 patients with fatal acute aortic dissection at autopsy and also about 200 patients who had resection of the ascending aorta because of acute medial dissection (type A, zone 0).[1-16]

What are the classic morphologic features of cardiovascular syphilis? Exactly what are these features in the first 10 or so years after the occurrence of the presenting syphilitic lesion is unclear to us. The patients with cardiovascular syphilis we have studied at necropsy or after excision of the syphilitic aorta had their primary syphilitic lesion 15 to 40 years earlier. Thus, the aorta in them was thicker than normal due to fibrous thickening of the intima and fibrous thickening of adventitia. The fibrous tissue in the adventitia contained focal clumps of plasma cells and lymphocytes and thickened vasa vasora. The media was not thickened but there was extensive focal loss of its elastic fibers and

occasionally inflammatory cells were present in this portion of the aorta. We have never seen *T. pallida* organisms in the aorta.

The classic morphologic lesion of acute aortic dissection is well known. A discrete intimal-medial tear is present (most commonly in the ascending portion and next most commonly in the descending thoracic aorta). The dissection is present in the media, usually in its outer portion, and neither the intima nor the adventitia is thickened. The media most commonly is normal before the onset of the dissection.[8]

Thus, aortic dissection is a medial disease and cardiovascular syphilis in a pan-aortic wall disease. Syphilis leads to medial scars which prevent propagation of the dissection and therefore make dissection an incredibly rare event in persons with cardiovascular syphilis. Indeed, cardiovascular syphilis might be viewed as a protective against the occurrence of aortic dissection.

As mentioned, the present case is the only one we have encountered in 60 years despite having a wide experience with both cardiovascular syphilis and aortic dissection.[1-16]

There have appeared, however, publications describing aortic dissection and cardiovascular syphilis in the same patient. Weiss[17] in 1938 described a 61-year-old woman who had an "old" saccular aneurysm at the aortic isthmus. The ascending and transverse portions of the aorta were normal. Histologic examination of the wall of the aneurysm disclosed "...endarteritis with thickening of the adventitia...consistent with a syphilitic process." The blood Wasserman and Hinton tests were positive. Bland and Castleman[18] in 1941 described a 47-year-old man with an earlier penile lesion, positive blood Hinton reaction, who had "...stellate scarring and linear tree barking..." in the tubular portion of aorta and its arch and a transverse intimal-medial

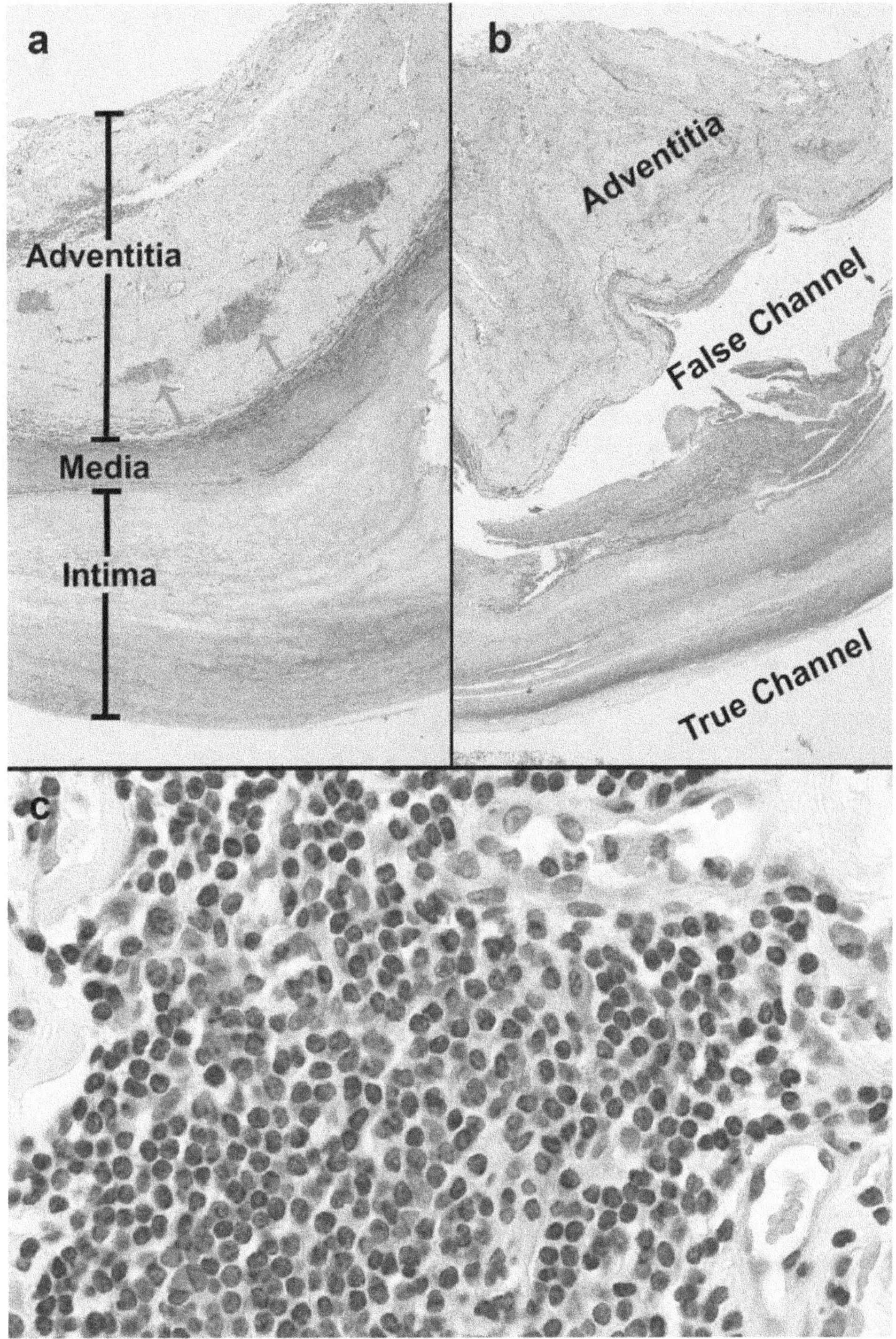

Figure 3. Shown here are photomicrographs of the ascending aorta in the patient described. a A section of the aorta showing the adventitia, the media, and the intima. The intima and adventitia are greatly thickened by fibrous tissue and the media, although not thickened, has lost most of its elastic fibers. Clumps of cells shown in c are designated by the arrows in the adventitia in a. b Section of aorta; the false channel is in the very outer media. The adventitia again is quite thick. c A close up of some of the cells designated by the arrow in a.

tear about 2 cm cephalad to the sino-tubular junction. "The dissection had not ascended above the point of intimal tear, stopping short at the point where the syphilitic aortitis became evident." The authors indicated ". . . that the syphilitic scarring prevented the distal extension of the dissection." These were insightful comments. Other cases of both cardiovascular syphilis and aortic dissection have been described but the descriptions of the cardiovascular syphilis were inadequate to confirm its presence.[19]

## Declaration of interests

The authors declare that they have no known competing financial interests or personal relationships that could have appeared to influence the work reported in this paper.


1. Roberts WC. Aortic dissection: Anatomy, consequences, and causes. *Am Heart J* 1981;101:195–214.
2. Warnes CA. Kirkmen PM, Roberts WC. Aortic dissection in more than one family member. *Am J Cardiol* 1985;55:236–238.
3. Roberts WC. Statler LF, Wallace RB. Hemodynamic confirmation of peripheral pulmonary stenosis caused by aortic dissection. *Am J Cardiol* 1989;63:1418–1420.
4. Roberts CS. Roberts WC. Aortic dissection with the entrance tear in transverse aorta: Analysis of 12 autopsy patients. *Ann Thor Surg* 1990;50:762–766.
5. Roberts CS, Roberts WC. Dissection of the aorta associated with congenital malformation of the aortic valve. *J Am Coll Cardiol* 1991;17:712–716.
6. Roberts CS, Roberts WC. Aortic dissection with the entrance tear in the descending thoracic aorta: Analysis of 40 necropsy patients. *Ann Surg* 1991;213:356–358.
7. Roberts CS, Roberts WC. Combined thoracic aortic dissection and abdominal aortic fusiform aneurysm. *Ann Thor Surg* 1991;52:537–540.
8. Roberts WC, Vowels TJ, Ko JM, Guileyardo JM. Acute aortic dissection with tear in ascending aorta not diagnosed until necropsy or operation (for another condition) and comparison to similar cases receiving proper operative therapy. *Am J Cardiol* 2012;110:728–735.
9. Roberts WC, Kapoor P, Main ML, Guileyardo JM. Acute aortic dissection with intussusception of the partition between the true and false channels leading to near total aortic occlusion (true aortic stenosis). *Am J Cardiol* 2017;119:340–344.
10. Roberts WC, Ko JM, Vowels TJ. Natural history of syphilitic aortitis. *Am J Cardiol* 2009;104:1578–1587.
11. Roberts WC, Bose R, Ko JM, Henry AC, Hamman BL. Identifying cardiovascular syphilis at operation. *Am J Cardiol* 2009;104:1588–1594.
12. Roberts WC, Lensing FD, Kourlis H Jr, Ko JM. Newberry JW. Smerud MJ, Burton EC, Hebeler RF Jr.. Full blown cardiovascular syphilis with aneurysm of the innominate artery. *Am J Cardiol* 2009;104:1595–1600.
13. Roberts WC, Vowels TJ, Kitchens BL, Ko JM, Filardo G, Henry AC, Hamman BL, Matter GJ, Hebeler RF Jr. Aortic medial elastic fiber loss in acute ascending aortic dissection. *Am J Cardiol* 2011;108:1639–1644.
14. Barbin CM, Weissenborn MR. Ko JM, Guileyardo JE, Roberts WC. Computed tomographic and morphologic features of syphilis of the aorta. *Am J Cardiol* 2015;116:1311–1314.
15. Roberts WC, Kondapalli N. Operative recognition of syphilis of the aorta. *Am J Cardiol* 2018;122:898–904.
16. Roberts WC, Moore AJ, Roberts CS. Syphilitic aortitis: Still a current common cause of aneurysm of the tubular portion of ascending aorta. *Cardiovasc Pathol* 2020;46:107175.
17. Weiss S. Dissecting aneurysm of the aorta. *N Eng J Med* 2009;218:512–517.
18. Mallory TB. Cabot case 27302 - (Bland EF, and Castleman B). Dissecting aneurysm of the aorta with rupture into pericardium. *N Eng J Med* 1941;225:155–159.
19. Flaxman N. Dissecting aneurysm of the aorta. *Am Heart J* 1942:654–664.

# Diagnosing aortic syphilis

Charles S. Roberts, MD[a,b], and William C. Roberts, MD[b,c,d]

[a]Department of Cardiac Surgery, Baylor University Medical Center, Dallas, Texas; [b]Baylor Scott & White Heart and Vascular Institute, Dallas, Texas; [c]Department of Internal Medicine, Baylor University Medical Center, Dallas, Texas; [d]Department of Pathology, Baylor University Medical Center, Dallas, Texas

**ABSTRACT**

Described herein is a morbidly obese 57-year-old man with an aneurysm involving the tubular portion of the aorta. Examination of the wall of the operatively resected aneurysm disclosed classic findings of aortic syphilis, a condition that clearly has not disappeared. If there is an aneurysm involving the tubular portion of the ascending aorta in the absence of aortic dissection or involvement of the sinuses of Valsalva, the most likely diagnosis is aortic syphilis. In these circumstances, the serologic test for syphilis is often negative.

**KEYWORDS** Aortic aneurysm; aortic operation; aortic syphilis

The patient, either a man or a woman, is >50 years of age, usually asymptomatic, may or may not have a precordial murmur, and possesses a normal-sized heart, but the area of the ascending aorta on the chest radiograph is enlarged. An echocardiogram and/or computed tomographic image shows the tubular portion of the aorta to be dilated without evidence of aortic dissection, the sinuses of Valsalva to be of normal size, and focal calcific deposits may or may not be present in the aneurysmal wall. The serologic test for syphilis may or may not be reactive. This scenario is the characteristic picture of the patient with aortic syphilis.[1–3] Such a case is described herein.

## CASE DESCRIPTION

A 57-year-old asymptomatic, obese (body mass index 40.5 kg/m$^2$) woman on routine checkup was found to have a soft precordial murmur; a chest radiograph and an echocardiogram showed a dilated ascending aorta (involving the tubular portion only). These findings led to her referral to Baylor University Medical Center's Aortic Clinic, where a computed tomographic image confirmed the fusiform aneurysm involving the tubular portion of the ascending aorta, its maximal diameter being 5.1 cm. The left ventricular ejection fraction was 55% to 60%, and the left ventricular cavity was of normal size. The electrocardiogram was normal. A serologic test for syphilis was negative. The aortic aneurysm was replaced with a 30-mm graft. Her postoperative course was uneventful. The operatively excised aorta is shown in *Figures 1 and 2*, and photomicrographs of portions of the aortic media are shown in *Figure 3*.

## DISCUSSION

Aortic syphilis has not disappeared.[1–4] It remains a major cause of aneurysm of the tubular portion of the aorta.[4] The process begins at the sinotubular junction, thus sparing the walls of the sinuses of Valsalva. Although on occasion the syphilitic process may involve one or more arteries arising from the arch and also the descending thoracic aorta, the process never involves the abdominal aorta (because there are no vaso vasora in this portion of the aorta). The wall of the aneurysm is 100% involved by the syphilitic process or nearly so. The aneurysm, thus, is fusiform, but on occasion one or more saccular aneurysms may arise from the wall of the fusiform aneurysm.

The histologic features of the aneurysmal wall are characteristic. All three layers of the wall are involved in the process. The adventitia is thickened by fibrous tissue containing focal collections of lymphocytes and plasmacytes. The walls of the vaso vasora are thicker than normal and their lumens are narrowed. (The latter appears to be responsible for the focal scarring of the media and the destruction of many of its elastic fibers. Sometimes the inflammatory process in the

**Corresponding author:** Charles S. Roberts, MD, 621 N. Hall Street, Suite 120, Dallas, TX 75226 (e-mail: Charles.Roberts@BSWHealth.org)

The authors report no funding or conflicts of interest.

Received June 13, 2022; Accepted July 18, 2022.

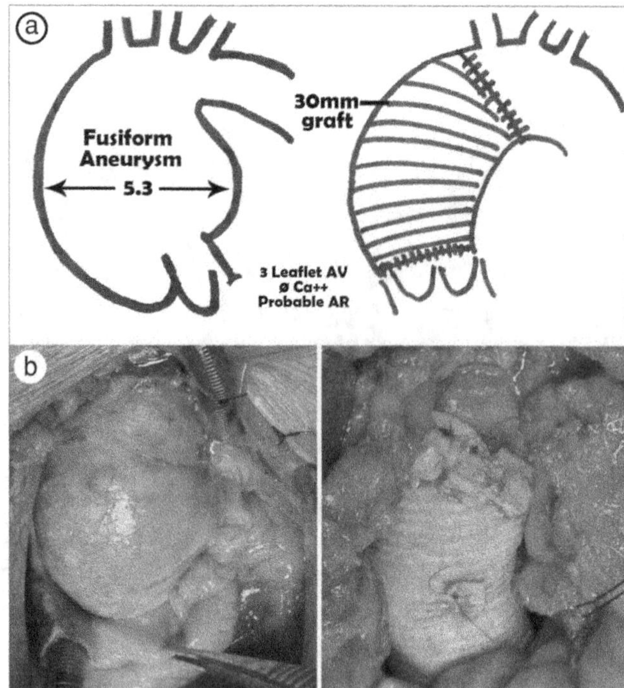

Figure 1. (a) Diagram of the aortic aneurysm before and after operative therapy. (b) View of the dilated ascending aorta before and after its replacement.

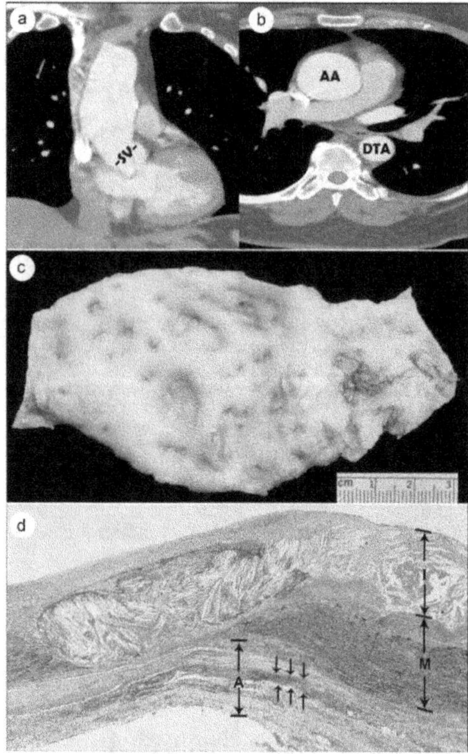

Figure 2. View of the aortogram showing the (a, b) dilated tubular portion of the aorta. The sinus of Valsalva (SV) is of normal size. AA indicates ascending aorta; DTA, descending thoracic aorta. (c) Opened aorta showing the extensive fibrous and calcific deposits on the intimal surface. The circumference of the aorta is 16 cm and, when intact, the diameter is 5.1 cm. (d) Photomicrograph of the wall of the fusiform aneurysm showing large collections of cholesterol clefts in the intima (I) and destroyed part of the media (M). The adventitia (A) is thickened by fibrous tissue within which are collections of lymphocytes and plasmacytes (small arrows). Movat stain, ×20.

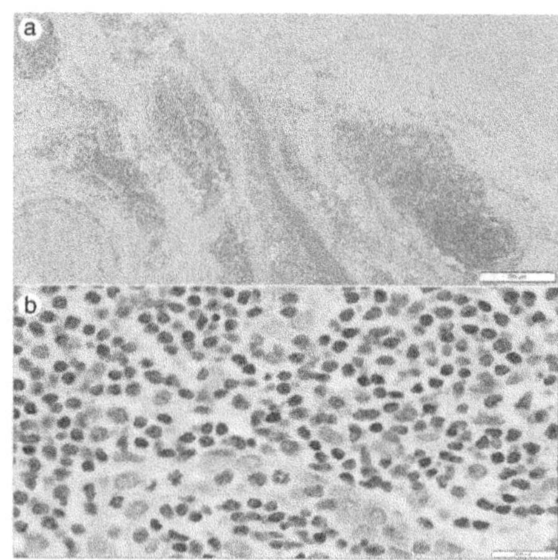

Figure 3. Photomicrographs of portions of the aortic media showing (a) large clumps of lymphocytes and plasmacytes and (b) a close-up of cells in the clumps. Hematoxylin-eosin stains, × 20 (a) and ×1000 (b).

adventitia extends into the media, which is not thickened by the process.) The intima is thickened mainly by fibrous tissue, often with focal calcific deposits. The consequence of this process is that the wall of the aorta is thicker than normal, but because of the disappearance of many elastic fibers in the media, the wall is weaker than normal, leading to the aneurysmal dilation. The presence of the scar tissue in the media essentially prevents the occurrence of aortic dissection in these patients.[5]

The main reason to diagnose syphilis as the cause of an aortic aneurysm is to prevent its massive expansion and rupture and to prompt the use of antibiotics to retard or prevent the occurrence of neurological syphilis. The unusual feature of the present case is the disposition in the aortic intima of *huge* quantities of calcific deposits.


1. Roberts WC, Ko JM, Vowels TJ. Natural history of syphilitic aortitis. *Am J Cardiol.* 2009;104(11):1578–1587. doi:10.1016/j.amjcard.2009.07.031.
2. Roberts WC, Bose R, Ko JM, Henry AC, Hamman BL. Identifying cardiovascular syphilis at operation. *Am J Cardiol.* 2009;104(11):1588–1594. doi:10.1016/j.amjcard.2009.06.071.
3. Roberts WC, Barbin CM, Weissenborn MR, Ko JM, Henry AC. Syphilis as a cause of thoracic aortic aneurysm. *Am J Cardiol.* 2015;116(8):1298–1303. doi:10.1016/j.amjcard.2015.07.030.
4. Roberts WC, Moore AJ, Roberts CS. Syphilitic aortitis: still a current common cause of aneurysm of the tubular portion of ascending aorta. *Cardiovasc Pathol.* 2020;46:107175. doi:10.1016/j.carpath.2019.107175.
5. Roberts WC, Roberts CS. Combined cardiovascular syphilis and type A acute aortic dissection. *Am J Cardiol.* 2022;168:159–162. doi:10.1016/j.amjcard.2021.10.040.